CONTENTS

WITNESSES

TELEMEDICINE: AN INFORMATION HIGHWAY TO SAVE LIVES

HEARING

BEFORE THE

SUBCOMMITTEE ON
INVESTIGATIONS AND OVERSIGHT

OF THE

COMMITTEE ON
SCIENCE, SPACE, AND TECHNOLOGY
U.S. HOUSE OF REPRESENTATIVES

ONE HUNDRED THIRD CONGRESS

SECOND SESSION

MAY 2, 1994

[No. 132]

Printed for the use of the
Committee on Science, Space, and Technology

U.S. GOVERNMENT PRINTING OFFICE

81–951 WASHINGTON : 1994

For sale by the U.S. Government Printing Office
Superintendent of Documents, Congressional Sales Office, Washington, DC 20402

ISBN 0-16-045817-X

COMMITTEE ON SCIENCE, SPACE, AND TECHNOLOGY

GEORGE E. BROWN, Jr., California, *Chairman*

MARILYN LLOYD, Tennessee
DAN GLICKMAN, Kansas
HAROLD L. VOLKMER, Missouri
RALPH M. HALL, Texas
DAVE McCURDY, Oklahoma
TIM VALENTINE, North Carolina
ROBERT G. TORRICELLI, New Jersey
RICK BOUCHER, Virginia
JAMES A. TRAFICANT, Jr., Ohio
JAMES A. HAYES, Louisiana
JOHN S. TANNER, Tennessee
PETE GEREN, Texas
JIM BACCHUS, Florida
TIM ROEMER, Indiana
ROBERT E. (BUD) CRAMER, Jr., Alabama
DICK SWETT, New Hampshire
JAMES A. BARCIA, Michigan
HERBERT C. KLEIN, New Jersey
ERIC FINGERHUT, Ohio
PAUL McHALE, Pennsylvania
JANE HARMAN, California
DON JOHNSON, Georgia
SAM COPPERSMITH, Arizona
ANNA G. ESHOO, California
JAY INSLEE, Washington
EDDIE BERNICE JOHNSON, Texas
DAVID MINGE, Minnesota
NATHAN DEAL, Georgia
ROBERT C. SCOTT, Virginia
XAVIER BECERRA, California
PETER W. BARCA, Wisconsin
BOBBY L. RUSH, Illinois

ROBERT S. WALKER, Pennsylvania[1]
F. JAMES SENSENBRENNER, Jr., Wisconsin
SHERWOOD L. BOEHLERT, New York
TOM LEWIS, Florida
HARRIS W. FAWELL, Illinois
CONSTANCE A. MORELLA, Maryland
DANA ROHRABACHER, California
STEVEN H. SCHIFF, New Mexico
JOE BARTON, Texas
DICK ZIMMER, New Jersey
SAM JOHNSON, Texas
KEN CALVERT, California
MARTIN R. HOKE, Ohio
NICK SMITH, Michigan
EDWARD R. ROYCE, California
ROD GRAMS, Minnesota
JOHN LINDER, Georgia
PETER BLUTE, Massachusetts
JENNIFER DUNN, Washington
BILL BAKER, California
ROSCOE G. BARTLETT, Maryland
VERNON J. EHLERS, Michigan

ROBERT E. PALMER, *Chief of Staff*
MICHAEL RODEMEYER, *Chief Counsel*
KATHRYN HOLMES, *Administrator*
DAVID D. CLEMENT, *Republican Chief of Staff*

SUBCOMMITTEE ON INVESTIGATIONS AND OVERSIGHT

JAMES A. HAYES, Louisiana, *Chairman*

JOHN S. TANNER, Tennessee
MARILYN LLOYD, Tennessee
DON JOHNSON, Georgia
SAM COPPERSMITH, Arizona

CONSTANCE A. MORELLA, Maryland
JOE BARTON, Texas
VERNON J. EHLERS, Michigan

[1] Ranking Republican Member.

TELEMEDICINE: AN INFORMATION HIGHWAY TO SAVE LIVES

MONDAY, MAY 2, 1994

HOUSE OF REPRESENTATIVES,
COMMITTEE ON SCIENCE, SPACE, AND TECHNOLOGY,
SUBCOMMITTEE ON INVESTIGATIONS AND OVERSIGHT,
Washington, DC.

The subcommittee met, pursuant to call, at 11:00 a.m. in Building 10, National Institute of Health, Hon. Jimmy Hayes (chairman of the subcommittee) presiding.

Mr. HAYES. Good morning. We are going to begin this session of the Committee on Science and Technology, the Investigation and Oversight Subcommittee, in an area that came to my attention because of a field hearing in Augusta on an unrelated subject involving approval times and delays in pharmaceuticals and in supplies. As a result of visiting the institution, I was so impressed with the technology being developed there and the potential for that technology throughout the remaining parts of the country and I later learned there are very interesting things done in several States, including my home State of Louisiana and for that reason thought this would be an appropriate site since you do so well coordinating research among, as I understand it, over 1700 universities and facilities around the Nation, that the message that some of these folks have to deliver would be well received, and we could have the ability to use your combined resources to perhaps further that process of dissemination.

It is also an area at the time there is so much discussion about health care that does not have the kind of visits to our office. There is no group left in America that has not been in our office saying here is what we like or don't like about this health care bill, and here is what we like and don't like about this other health care bill, and here is what we like and don't like generally. But the audience for research is not the same, so it doesn't elicit the same kinds of responses where the organized visits come in and say here is much more information on preventative care and on how some cost reduction can come about rather than increases, and here is some important information about what ought to be more available.

We are trying to help fill that void by hosting this so close to the Washington communities and reaching Members who do not serve on every committee related to health care, but ought to be hearing some of the things that are said here and ought to know more about some of the things that are done here at this site.

With that having been said, I am pleased to be here in the home of Ms. Morella, and would recognize her for her opening statement.

Mrs. MORELLA. Welcome to Bethesda, Maryland and the National Institutes of Health. Since we have an exciting set of witnesses today in a relatively short period, I am going to keep my opening remarks brief so that we can spend as much time assist as is necessary with our witnesses and their demonstrations. I want to extend my appreciation to you for holding today's hearing and for your leadership in recognizing the potential of telemedicine to improve the delivery of our Nation's health care.

I am also pleased to host today's subcommittee hearing here in Montgomery County. This is the district I am honored to represent. It is the home also to some of our Nation's most important Federal research laboratories, a major industrial sector and also home to a developing university presence, Montgomery County is considered one of our nation's leading high technology areas.

The Federal Government's scientific presence in Montgomery County includes the Food and Drug Administration, the National Institute of Standards and Technology as well as NIH. These critical agencies all play major roles in improving and maintaining our Nation's health and welfare. So, as we explore the issue of information technologies in the delivery of medical care, it seems only logical for us to be holding this hearing here at NIH.

As we know, NIH is the principal biomedical research agency of the Federal Government with its mission of pursuing knowledge to improve human health. I have had numerous opportunities to personally witness the fine work of our NIH employees, some of whom have joined us here today. These dedicated scientists, under the leadership of Dr. Varmus and Dr. Kirschstein have been asked to take on the enormous medical challenges that face the U.S. as we prepare for the new century. The research activities being conducted by NIH scientists are determining the current quality of our Nation's health care.

As a component of NIH, the National Library of Medicine serves as our Nation's chief medical information source. I am very proud of them. NLM is responsible for applying advanced technologies to the improvement of biomedical communications and has a leadership role in the development and application of telemedicine. I am pleased to welcome Dr. Lindberg, the Director of the National Library of Medicine to our subcommittee. Dr. Lindberg will let us know of the important telemedicine advances being made here at the National Library of Medicine.

Mr. Chairman, as Congress begins debate on reforming our Nation's health care system, telemedicine and health care technologies are becoming an important facet of that debate. The benefits of telemedicine can help improve the delivery of health care.

These benefits include immediate access to medical expertise regardless of the location of the patient and more timely diagnoses and treatment. In addition, telemedicine applications have demonstrated the great potential for significant health cost savings, as well as the ability to provide for high quality medical care to communities that don't have the medical experts and specialty services.

Now that telemedicine technology has been improved and is widely available and affordable, we need to investigate the full application and potential of this technology. So I am especially interested in hearing from our witnesses what Government can do to remove some of the barriers which stand in the way of wider deployment of telemedicine services.

I thank you, Mr. Chairman, and look forward to hearing from our witnesses.

Mr. HAYES. Thank you. Before our first panel we want to introduce Dr. Ruth Kirschstein, the Deputy Director of NIH.

STATEMENT OF DR. RUTH KIRSCHSTEIN, DEPUTY DIRECTOR, NATIONAL INSTITUTES OF HEALTH

Dr. KIRSCHSTEIN. Thank you. We want to welcome Congressman Hayes and Congresswoman Morella. We are very honored that you have chosen the NIH as the site for your field hearing on telemedicine.

On behalf of Dr. Varmus, I want to welcome you as well. As you begin this hearing, I can't help but recall that the person who put the "tele" part in telemedicine was very much involved in this county, Montgomery County. The inventor of the telephone, Alexander Graham Bell was deeply interested in the problems of the hearing impaired because his wife, Mabel, was deaf. The technology that Bell developed for the telephone was rapidly adapted to the hearing aid before the turn of the century, and I think you could call hearing aids a first example of telemedicine for they utilized in some small way telecommunications to improve health.

Today in harness with high performance computing, telecommunications technology is advancing with a speed matched only by that of biomedical research. There is no question that these new capabilities will have a profound effect on the speed with which new medical discoveries are formulated, communicated and translated into effective patient care.

A number of the units at NIH have programs that relate to such communications. As we speak here, the Division of Computer Research and Technology is having a symposium celebrating its 20th anniversary. You will hear soon from the other important part of NIH, the National Library of Medicine.

So we congratulate this subcommittee for its foresight in holding this hearing at the National Institutes of Health, the crossroads of the information superhighway and the biomedical research interchange. Once again, welcome and best wishes for a productive and illuminating hearing.

Thank you very much.

Mr. HAYES. Thank you.

Our first panel that I have the privilege to introduce is Dr. Lindberg, who is with the National Library of Medicine and the Chair of the High Performance Computing and Communications Initiative, and Dr. Helen Smits, Deputy Administrator of the Health Care Financing Administration. Dr. Dena Puskin of the Office of Rural Health Policy is delayed this morning, but will join us later and will be included in one of our subsequent panels.

One housekeeping statement for all witnesses—each statement will be a complete part of the record and, therefore, we would certainly ask and indeed encourage you not only to summarize some parts to express observations but need not fear whether you follow your written text in that that would be included, as well.

So if you hear comments from other witnesses that you would like to elaborate on, do so. We will keep the record so anyone who wishes to augment with additional information or resources, we are delighted to have that as an additional part of what becomes a permanent record and perhaps be of assistance to other people who want to look at this record for guidance on telemedicine and health care.

Dr. Lindberg, proceed in any manner you wish with your statement.

STATEMENT OF DR. DONALD A. B. LINDBERG, M.D., DIRECTOR, NATIONAL LIBRARY OF MEDICINE

Dr. LINDBERG. Thank you, Congressman Hayes. Thank you for offering us the opportunity to discuss this interesting topic. I appreciate your coming to NIH just as Dr. Kirschstein said. I should perhaps just telegraph my conclusions right at the outset of my brief remarks. I am very enthusiastic about the potential for telemedicine to improve our ability to care for people and to improve the quality of life in rural and frontier areas. And I am quite convinced that the time has come in which the technology will permit significant experiments and is perhaps even close at hand to completing that process. So I am definitely an enthusiast for this field.

Perhaps I should, as a good library-type speak a moment about definitions. What do we mean by "telemedicine"? It does matter a bit. I don't think it is a difficult term. I rather like the definition HRSA used in a recent grant solicitation. Telemedicine is the use of telecommunications for medical diagnosis and patient care. That seems reasonable to me.

NLM has a preexisting definition which we use as a guide to persons indexing the literature. Telemedicine is delivery of host services via remote telecommunications. This includes interactive consultative and diagnostic services. So people are reasonably in agreement on this.

I do point out that this is a pretty broad proposition. This is not a particular technology, a particular format, a particular piece of equipment or a particular set of diagnoses.

An even broader definition I heard last week at a Capitol Hill hearing—John Silva said it was providing medical information at a distance. That is certainly the root of all of these because the consultative and diagnostic services hinge upon more information. I am grateful to Dr. Kirschstein for her remarks and I feel that a tip of the hat to history is appropriate.

Twenty years ago NLM was collaborating with NASA on a series of satellites which allowed the Public Health Service doctors to see, if you will, patients in remote Alaskan villages. Over the years, there have been a number of such attempts at health care delivery and demonstrations using telecommunications technology. It worked rather well then. It was expensive, yet in spite of this early success, there are today only a few uses of communications for telemedicine that are so widespread that we would consider them to be conventional.

Among those would be use of cardiac telemetry by emergency response teams, and the automated interpretation of electrocardiograms that are transmitted by telephone lines. The latter I was working on myself back in the mid-1960s and it was fully operational on a statewide basis by 1968. That certainly is telemedicine.

The enthusiasm and interest in the field now I think probably stems mostly from the continuing awareness of the need to provide consultation in rural areas, really anywhere where medicine is needed. Each and every one of us would like I suppose telemedicine brought to us in an emergency wherever that emergency occurred, and we would like the consultation of whomever could help us best.

So the idea is certainly an old and appealing idea, but probably the reason for your hearing and the reason for the appropriateness of the interest is because the communications technology is now so effective and, as you suggested, one of my other activities is on behalf of the White House Science Office to conduct a high performance computing communications initiative.

One of its major activities is investigating feasibility and design of high speed communication lines, including international centers on NREN the Federal high speed back bone. The goal there is to provide a billion bits per second coast-to-coast available to whomever needs it at whatever time it is needed in a reliable fashion, initially through lines which are created by government programs, but as soon as possible, and it is coming quite soon, on a commercial basis by competing vendors.

Now, that essentially means that there is enough band width to do the experiments that everyone is interested in doing, to see the patient, to see the patient in color, to see the patient in high resolution, to see the patient move if necessary. And these were not imaginable 25 years ago. But it does not mean that I must say a bit about the status of Internet. It is the biggest such network the world has ever seen. There are roughly one-and-a-half million computers on the network. There are 15,000 sub-networks that are part of Internet, some networks are statewide networks, such as the State of Texas.

So they overlap. There are a thousand universities, a thousand high schools, a hundred countries. So it is very big, but it probably still only touches 1 or 2 percent of our population, not by design but because it is an experimental network, a research and education network. So for telemedicine to come into its full flower, we would like to imagine that the entire population, not 2 percent but 100 percent would have access to these services when required.

Again, because I know that the time is limited, I do want to give a suggestion to you of a way to look at telemedicine. To me it falls into three parts: one is aids to cognition and decision-making; secondly is remote sensing; three is collaborative arrangements for management of patients at a distance.

The first, aids to cognition and decision-making is the most information-dependent. That is how the National Library of Medicine became so firmly committed to this field, because there are 6 million occasions a year in which our computer is directly accessed by doctors and we know by survey that half those occasions involve the treatment of individual patients.

There is software such that a doctor can make the call himself or herself. There are also networks of medical libraries and medical librarians so that if one is lucky enough to have that professional assistance, the call can be made by an expert searcher. There are 4,000 libraries in the network to provide copies of the material as required. In the new network it is possible to send digital copies of the pages involved.

So we know from all these studies that providing information at the time and place of medical decision-making is a major part of telemedicine.

In addition to just plain scientific information, there are computer programs that combine the knowledge of particular medical subjects with inferencing mechanisms that enable the program to solve a medical problem, to make a diagnosis, to critique treatment. These are called "expert systems". There are very few, perhaps less than a dozen that are worthwhile, but they are all developed at individual universities and are part of Internet and available increasingly countrywide. Without exception, all of those have had NIH support over the last 20 years. They are all scientific systems.

Remote sensing would include EKGs, but also now images and that require a whole lot more bandwidth. I want to give a couple of examples. The National Cancer Institute at NIH is working with GE to develop a system that will allow the management, compression and transmission of 3–D MRI images of the breast. The point of that examination is early detection of breast cancer. They are hopeful it will do that.

If that were the case, you would want to transmit the data to a central point where a computer could do the interpretation and provide that as a central service. First you have to know it is worthwhile.

In a similar vein, NLM has a project involving some 30,000 x-rays. These are part of the health and nutrition and evaluation study in which the interpretation of the X-rays is made [1] centrally and the films are held locally throughout the country and not as part of a national study, a radiological study of arthritis and disease of the bone and joint. There is a visible human project that NLM supports where the University of Colorado as contractors is producing a data set which will be three dimensional, an entire structure of an adult male and female, histology, magnetic resonance imaging and CAT scanning, so a milestone and a means of standardizing the transmission of all images anatomical is available on the Internet.

Just to mention other NIH efforts, the National Center for Research Resources funds telemicroscopy projects in which you can control an experiment across the country. The collaborative patient management issues are probably the most important. Obviously, those involve arrangements among people and institutions. Those are harder in a lot of ways than electronics. When NLM last year announced it was interested in supporting high performance computer and communications projects in the health sciences, the largest number of proposals received was for test bed networks and for collaborative technology for real time management of patients.

---

[1] Dr. Lindberg wants to delete "made centrally and the films are held locally throughout the country and not as part of a national study, a" and insert "to be performed at a number of different sites in this."

As a result, we have funded now city-wide networks in Indianapolis and Chicago; area-wide, western Pennsylvania; statewide, Iowa and West Virginia; and a network for underserved rural areas in Kansas.

Jumping ahead, there is another set of research grants that my institution has funded for the last 10 years called integrated advanced information management systems and some 20 schools have been funded over the years to support planning for information systems across the entire institution. You can imagine 10 years ago—it was really 12 years ago when the idea arose, that was an advanced idea.

Now we realize they should be planning for an entire region, States, and interestingly enough, in the last round we just funded an institution at Louisiana State University in Louisiana, your home State. This is not only a single institutional grant, but it proposes to link together 36 other schools and medical institutions statewide. So this is working on that collaborative infrastructure that makes it possible to actually do the telemedicine.

There are a couple of issues to be mentioned. Will the communications technology get to everywhere? That is one issue. We open the paper every day to hear about new fleets of communication satellites proposed and greater band widths, so perhaps that will take care of itself.

The second issue, the social concerns, will the collaborative arrangements get made? There we take into account licensing across State boundaries, liability issues. I think those will be described perhaps by Dr. Sanders.

An issue that is of great concern to the White House perhaps is privacy and confidentiality of computerized records. Your colleague, Representative Condit, has introduced a bill that would establish a uniform Federal code for handling computer-based records. Something like that probably is desirable, we believe.

In any event, the technology of user authentication, data encryption and such that are part of the HPCC initiative probably will be used in the computerized patient records, but the arrangements that the patient wants are yet unclear. In other words, the point is not to lock up the record and make it absolutely unattainable. Quite the reverse. Each of us wants the record to be highly available if we get in trouble and want treatment.

The last issue I should mention is the economics. What will this do to costs? It seems quite likely to me that one could show significant cost savings in the treatment of individual patients by application of telemedicine systems, yet what would be the ultimate financial effect on the overall health care bill as more and more patients are served.

I think one doesn't have enough information to answer that question yet and it seems to me an appropriate question for the Federal Government to pursue very actively.

Telemedicine programs exist in a number of other Federal agencies, including HCFA and the Office of Rural Health of HRSA. Also, the National Institute of Mental Health supports research in telepsychiatry, amazingly enough. I wouldn't have thought that was workable, but they seem to think it is worth trying.

The Indian Health Service is beginning to support some telemedicine projects at University of Arizona, specifically. It is hooked up to Internet. The Rural Electrification Administration has a grant program. NASA has a grant—sponsors a program known as Telemedicine Demonstration Projects that link U.S. medical schools with the Johnson Space Center and with a hospital in Moscow and that uses telepathology and a teleradiology system developed by DOD.

There is an interesting set of activities within the Federal Government. I should mention the VA. Some 600 facilities and 22,000 miles of quite advanced digital networking. They are starting to experiment with teleconsultation, including images, voice and EKG.

NTIA, the National Telecommunications and Information Agency, in Commerce sponsors a program that this year will award $26 million of matching grants to interconnect schools, libraries and hospitals and government agencies.

Lastly, the DOE has done important research work in projects relating to medical images. Their supercomputers are used in experiments and cancer therapy planning. I have to say this is not an exhaustive catalogue of Federal agencies providing such support. Such a catalogue doesn't exist and probably I have overlooked some and perhaps important agencies, but I want you to know that a lot is going on, a lot is interesting and high quality.

I don't see any problem of duplication or conflicts at all. I think for the moment it is complementary and quite important and I welcome your interest in the area.

Thank you.

[The prepared statement of Dr. Lindberg follows:]

Hearing of the House Science, Space, and
Technology Committee

Subcommittee on
Investigations and Oversight

National Institutes of Health
May 2, 1994

Testimony from Donald A. B. Lindberg, M.D.
Director, National Library of Medicine

Chairman Hayes and members of the Committee.

I appreciate this opportunity to tell you about telemedicine and the several programs of the National Institutes of Health that bear on it.

Telemedicine techniques usually are associated with direct patient care, but they can also be used for remote control of research instruments. The latter is of direct interest to NIH. In addition, much basic research in medical informatics, image acquisition, visualization, and mathematical modeling has been supported by NIH institutes. I will not describe today all the background or infrastructure work. Today I will mention briefly work that is directly aimed at telemedicine applications.

Terminology need not concern us here--I believe the simple definition of telemedicine that the Health Resources and Services Administration recently adopted in its grants solicitation is quite serviceable. Telemedicine is the use of telecommunications for medical diagnosis and patient care. You will hear from a HRSA representative today.

Telemedicine is not new. Twenty years ago the National Library of Medicine was using NASA satellites to allow Public Health Service doctors to "see" patients in remote Alaska villages. Over the years there have been a number of health care delivery experiments and demonstrations using the telecommunications technology available.

In spite of this work, there are today only a few uses of communications for telemedicine that are so widespread as to be considered "conventional." Among these would be the use of cardiac telemetry by emergency response teams and the automated interpretation of electrocardiograms transmitted by phone lines.

Today's interest in telemedicine is fueled by society's fervor for communications technology and, especially, the "information superhighway." And, indeed, much is possible now that wasn't even imaginable 20 years ago. Economical high-speed computers and fiberoptic digital communications technology advances have paved the way for a rich variety of medical services that can be provided in a distance-independent fashion.

To illustrate this point, I would like arbitrarily to divide telemedicine into three areas: aids to cognition and decision-making, remote sensing, and collaborative arrangements for the management of patients at a distance.

Aids to cognition and decision-making

Medicine is surely one of the most information-intensive professions. So productive is America's research that staying abreast of new life-saving knowledge is extremely difficult for physicians. This is the reason for the rapid growth and widespread popularity of a telecommunications program knows as "Grateful Med," developed by the National Library of Medicine. This program allows easy and inexpensive access to the Library's immense databases by members of a network of 75,000 health professionals in the United States and Canada. A recent study of physicians who use these databases revealed that the information gained frequently influences for the better how a doctor diagnoses and treats a patient. The 4,000 member institutions of the National Network of Libraries of Medicine not only promote the use of Grateful Med among health professionals, but also provide access to the full text of journal articles and other medical literature.

Online databases, however, are only one aspect of telemedicine applied to medical decision-making. For example, there are computer programs that combine knowledge of a particular medical subject with inferencing mechanisms that enable the program to help solve a medical problem. Such a program in the area of rheumatology has been developed at the NLM and has been field tested in various parts of the country. Telemedicine might make an "expert rheumatologist" available for consultation whenever and wherever needed.

The NIH, in a collaborative effort among the Division of Computer Research and Technology, Clinical Center, and National Cancer Institute, is implementing a prototype high-speed network, capable of supporting multimedia communication for medical research and education, on the NIH campus. A supercomputer will be connected to the network that will use the power of parallel computing methods for the computationally intensive calculations that are required for radiation therapy planning. Special-purpose medical workstations will be deployed as nodes to the prototype network in other selected domains on the campus.

Remote sensing

The second area is that of remote sensing. Images, of course, are extremely important in the practice of medicine. It is only recently that our long distance telecommunications capabilities have been improved to the point where we can send large and complex clinical images to colleagues across the country. Thus, many of today's state of the art experiments include transmitting Computer Tomography, Magnetic Resonance, photomicrographs for tissue diagnosis (telepathology), and digitized x-ray images (teleradiology). In a telemammography project at NIH, the

National Cancer Institute is working with General Electric to develop a system that will allow the management, compression, and transmission of 3-D images of the breast.

As another example, the National Library of Medicine has created a digital radiology system that provides access via the Internet to 30,000 digital x-rays. These images support epidemiologic research into the incidence of bone and arthritic disorders in the U.S. population. Also, the NLM is assembling an image database that will comprise a comprehensive collection of 2-D and 3-D images of complete human beings. The Visible Human Project, as it is called, will form the basis of a new generation of workstations for teaching human anatomy and help to create standards for exchanging clinical images over high-speed networks.

NIH's National Center for Research Resources has funded a telemicroscopy project to explore the feasibility of employing computers to operate an electron microscope from a remote location, using a high-speed network for transmitting commands to the microscope and receiving the images. By making such complex and costly instruments available from a remote site we can more efficiently conduct research and deliver health care.

Collaborative patient management

There is great current interest in using telemedicine for the third area I wish to mention--the management of patients. Smooth digital motion pictures are now becoming feasible and systems being developed will test 2-way "workstation video" for interactions between doctors for obtaining specialty consultation. Telemedicine systems also allow physicians to observe and discuss symptoms with patients who are far away. For example, a recent study in Parkinson's disease showed that doctors observing movement disorders of patients via interactive video were able to make adjustments to medication dosage with the same accuracy as physicians who evaluated the patients in person. Some studies show that rather than being alienated by video technology, patients appreciate being able to see and hear their doctor while in the comfort of their home.

When the National Library of Medicine last year announced that it was interested in supporting High Performance Computing and Communications projects in the health sciences, the greatest number of proposals received was for testbed networks and for collaborative technology for real-time treatment of patients. As a result, NLM has funded city-wide networks (Indianapolis, Chicago), area-wide (Western Pennsylvania), state-wide (Iowa and West Virginia), and networks for underserved rural areas (in Oregon and Kansas). The awards total $27 million over 3 years.

The first award, to a consortium of West Virginia institutions, is titled "Collaborative Technology for Real-Time Treatment of Patients." We hope to learn from it how primary care doctors and specialists in different settings--rural and urban--can collaborate in real time to treat patients using electronic patient records and knowledge from distributed sites.

There is also an NLM program to help large medical institutions devise methods for integrating the many diverse sources of computerized information. The Integrated Advanced Information Management Systems program ("IAIMS") has over the last decade supported a number of successful systems (for example, Columbia and Georgetown Universities) that are able to tie together electronically such disparate data sources as patient records, admissions, x-ray, and pharmacy. A particularly ambitious IAIMS project, not just for one institution, but to link together 36 schools and other medical institutions statewide, has just been funded in Louisiana, based on the LSU Medical Center.

Broad issues facing telemedicine

I would like now to discuss briefly several crucial issues that will ultimately determine to what extent society will benefit from the promise of telemedicine.

The first is the state of the communications technology infrastructure available to us. I've listed this as an issue, but in reality it is likely to be a non-issue. Anyone who scans the daily papers is aware that the information infrastructure grows ever more robust. There we read of projected fleets of communications satellites, ever greater bandwidth allowing ever more information to be transmitted ever more rapidly, and of wider access to more people--even K-12 access to the Internet. In short, all those things I have discussed that we hope to do in telemedicine are now possible, or very soon likely will be, within the current state of communications technology.

The second issue concerns the social aspects of telemedicine. This is a genuine issue, with problems that need to be addressed. One of these problems is the lack of agreed-on standards for information exchange. We desperately need widely accepted standards for representing and communicating medical and billing information. A related problem is that, for telemedicine systems involving licensed health professionals from different states, differing state licensure and accreditation requirements are an additional complication. Also, what will be the malpractice implications as these physicians, remote from each other and remote from the sources of information on which they rely, use telemedicine and various computerized aids in their practices?

Another social issue is the concern for privacy and confidentiality of computerized records. This is a subject that the Congress will soon be taking up, since Representative Gary A. Condit (D-CA) earlier this year introduced the Fair Health Information Practices Act of 1994. This bill would establish a uniform Federal code for handling individually identifiable health information that is used in the health treatment and payment processes. As the Department has testified, patients will be frank only if we can assure them that we will honor the confidentiality of their records. This will permit us not only to provide the best treatment, but to interrupt the spread of communicable disease and to gather accurate information for research about disease.

Of course, the need for secure and confidential electronic communication is not confined to medical care, as the recent debate over the "clipper chip" demonstrates. I believe that much of the technology created in the defense and intelligence communities, and financial systems, can and will be incorporated into any telemedicine systems that are widely deployed. User authentication, data encryption, and other technologies are important components of the High Performance Computing and Communications initiative that will be incorporated into future medical systems. There are a number of ongoing projects to develop a "Computerized Patient Record," and privacy concerns are being addressed in these efforts.

The third issue is economic--how do the costs of telemedicine compare with the benefits to be gained. This is an area in which we have insufficient data from this or alternative investment strategies. It seems quite likely that one could show significant cost savings in the treatment of individual patients by the application of telemedine systems. Yet, what would be the ultimate financial effect upon the entire health care bill as more such patients were served, isn't known today. I believe that an important role for the Federal Government is to investigate the potential savings to society by applying telecommunications and other High Performance Computing and Communications technology to health care in a testbed mode. There is an evaluation component in the recent telemedicine awards from NLM that I mentioned earlier, and I am hopeful that we will learn something from these and future studies.

Other federal agencies

There has never been a comprehensive survey of Federal agencies to determine what telemedicine projects are being supported. I know of several within the

Department of Health and Human Services, in addition to the Health Care Financing Administration from which you are also hearing today. The Office of Rural Health Policy of the Health Resources and Services Administration has a program of grants to investigate whether telemedicine can improve access to health services for rural residents and reduce the isolation of rural practitioners. It is expected that eight awards totaling $4 million will be made this year.

The Indian Health Service, with widespread health care facilities, is also beginning to support some telemedicine projects. In the short term, a demonstration project, with the University of Arizona, is being set up to employ the Internet as a medium for telemedicine communications. Longer term, the IHS is interested in developing a teleradiology capability.

There are other Federal agencies involved with telemedicine. The Rural Electrification Administration has announced a project grants program to support the use of telecommunications and computer networks to provide educational and medical benefits to people living in rural areas. Hospitals and medical centers are among those qualified to apply. $10 million was awarded to 28 applicants late in 1993. Another $10 million will be awarded to successful applicants in 1994.

The National Aeronautics and Space Administration sponsors a program known as the Telemedicine Demonstration Project that links four U.S. medical centers and the Johnson Space Center with the Clinical Hospital of the Medical Department of the Ministry of the Interior in Moscow. This project incorporates state of the art medical technologies, including a telepathology and teleradiology system developed by the Department of Defense.

The Department of Veterans Affairs has in recent years developed a sophisticated information infrastructure of hardware, software, hospital information systems, and a wide area network connecting its many hospital sites to support the exchange of medical data. The VA network, which connects over 600 major facilities, consists of 23,000 miles of fully digital optical fiber network that carries 21 gigabytes of data per month. Teleconsultation--including images, voice, electrocardiogram signals, and patient reports--is undergoing initial testing using the network.

The National Telecommunications and Information Administration (Department of Commerce) sponsors a program that will award $26 million this year in matching grants to interconnect schools, libraries, hospitals, and government agencies. Telemedicine and health care informatics are also being supported by NTIA grants in 1994.

Laboratories in the Department of Energy have been involved in a number of projects related to medical imaging. Initiatives include extracting information from images, data fusion of PET, CAT, and x-ray images and automated artificial intelligence projects involving remote transmission. In addition, efforts to improve treatment planning for cancer therapy are being studied using supercomputers at DOE laboratories. The work is occurring at Sandia, Lawrence Berkley, Lawrence Livermore, and Los Alamos laboratories.

This is not an exhaustive catalog of Federal agencies providing such support. Such a catalog does not exist and there are no doubt other agencies that have also supported relevant work at one time or another.

Mr. Chairman, I thank you for this opportunity to talk about telemedicine. It will assume ever greater importance as the National Information Infrastructure evolves and we seek to employ its tremendous capacity to the improvement of the Nation's health. I would be glad to answer any questions.

Mr. HAYES. Thank you very much.

From our experience we retain questions until the end of the entire panel.

Dr. Smits, please proceed.

STATEMENT OF DR. HELEN L. SMITS, M.D., DEPUTY ADMINISTRATOR, HEALTH CARE FINANCING ADMINISTRATOR

Dr. SMITS. Thank you, Mr. Chairman. I will be brief. Thank you for inviting me. It is a real pleasure to be here.

I first became involved with telemedicine last fall when the Rural Caucus approached the Health Care Financing Administration and asked us to consider the issues of Medicare coverage for these services. HCFA does not specifically dictate to States on the kinds of decisions they might make about something like telemedicine, but obviously if we decide within Medicare to cover it, then most States would follow in coverage for Medicaid.

For coverage purposes, it is probably useful to remention the definitions, not that they are particularly different. We really make a very sharp distinction between the use of telecommunications to transmit images which are traditionally interpreted in the absence of the patient, and transmission of either interactive information or non-interactive information which essentially substitutes for the person-to-person interaction that goes on between a consultant and a patient.

In the first group, you have EKG's, scans, radiology, including both images that start out as analog and have to be digitized and images that are digital to begin with. We have no restrictions in Medicare. We don't tell you how you have to get your hands on a x-ray or EKG or scan.

The only way Medicare would become involved in defining payment for telemedicine in the image area would be if questions were raised about quality or appropriateness. As far as we can tell that work has evolved with a great deal of thought to the quality of the image. Where I came from in Connecticut; most systems that were reading x-rays over teleradiology, reread them at some point with the hard copy. We are conservative in Connecticut.

I gather in other parts of the country radiologists reread a certain percentage or only those films they are concerned about. We know Medicare paid for those services and support that. As we move along, we may issue guidelines in terms of quality and there are some areas where the American College of Radiology tells us the image is not good enough.

If that is the case, we will include that in our guidance.

The issue I would like to talk about today is the use of telemedicine technology to substitute for actual transport of the patient or the consulting physician. I have had the great privilege of visiting several sites to look at telemedicine, usually from the central part of the site. I hope as the Spring wears on now and travel is better to also travel through some of the rural sites so I can talk directly with rural practitioners.

I have been very impressed with what I have seen in places like Lubbock, Texas and Augusta, Georgia where an academic health center makes the full range of its specialists available over telemedicine linkage to rural practitioners.

One of the interesting characteristics of most of those consultations is that they usually involve a new pattern of practice; that is the primary care practitioner sits with the patient through the consultation, partly to be able to provide additional information, and partly to do whatever sophisticated physical exam the consultant wishes. The result is that the consultants communicate with the patient and with the primary care doctor or primary care nurse practitioner or physician's assistant; these two things that used to go on separately now go on at once. That is an interesting change in practice and one we are very interested in evaluating.

Despite my personal enthusiasm for these projects, we also have to acknowledge that there have been only about 2,000 telemedicine consultations done in the last year in this country. That is an estimate done by one of the practitioners. But we certainly don't have the information on which we could base Medicare coverage rules.

Medicare does prohibit the payment to a consultant if the consultant has no personal interaction with the patient. That is based on other situations and circumstances. But we wouldn't want to change the coverage rules specifically for telemedicine unless we knew very precisely what we were doing.

Some of our concerns are licensure and liability issues and hospital privilege issues. Hospital privilege is an important part of quality control and it is unclear how that is going to play out in some of these settings. There are also questions as to how much we should define the quality of the image.

My current bias is that rural sites ought to be encouraged to buy the least expensive system that will serve them. This is an area where you can get involved in the high technology pretty quickly. But a few thousand dollars difference in purchase price makes a big difference to a rural hospital. So it is important that we balance quality with affordability.

I think in the long run there are very important questions of patient acceptability. Patients seem to like it very much. It enhances their view of their primary care practitioner; they think it is glamorous. Often a person who has been seen on telemedicine arrives at the transfer hospital: "saying I am the television patient." I am not sure as it becomes more common that that will be as true.

Clearly, there are some kinds of consultation, I would think some kinds of psychiatric consultation, where patients would be very uncomfortable about the presence of anyone else at the consultation, which is often necessary technically, and about the presence of a tape that could be played back.

There are questions about direct doctor-patient use of telemedicine. I think that ought to be explored.

Finally, there are very tricky questions of the potential these systems have for undercutting rather than supporting the very rural practitioners we want to bring more access. Rural practitioners well-linked to an academic center feel wonderful about the system. They feel supported. In every one of the consultations I have watched, the rural practitioner almost always knew what was going on.

They may have a few diagnostic wrinkles that they are not certain of, but they want help on management. Modern management of complicated patients tends to change fast. Someone who has handled a thousand critically ill babies in the last few years can tell the primary care practitioner things about how to care for the infants that are different, even though the practitioner knows that he has a critically ill child with an aspiration pneumonia and an electrolyte situation.

Practitioners feel great about that. One of the toughest things about rural practice in this country is the overwhelmingly complex patients you face, often on an emergency basis. Knowing there is someone willing to get on the television set and help you through it makes a big difference.

So what we would like to see at HCFA would be the creation of what we call pilot sites, sites where we could use medicare money to pay for consultation while collecting information about the range, appropriateness and acceptability of the service. We think that this is the best way to take the next step so that we can have good guidelines to use as we move forward to broader coverage. We also need at some point, to address the question of use of telemedicine in underserved urban as well as rural areas.

In closing, I would like to note that this has been a particularly interesting area for me because it is brand new to me and I have had a good chance to learn about it. Also I think it is an example of excellent interagency cooperation. As you know, a number of agencies have given capital grants to start up the systems. HRSA and the Rural Electrification Agency now have money for development. Commerce with some of the grants associated with the national information infrastructure has been particularly important in putting these systems in place. And HCFA is delighted to work with other agencies in terms of taking the next steps and exploring how the Government ought to pay for telemedicine in its own fee-for-service system.

We hope, in the meantime, that private payers, especially managed care payers, will adopt the system, pay for it and provide us with their information about what they think is a reasonable and appropriate use of the service.

Thank you very much.

[The prepared statement of Dr. Smits follows:]

DEPARTMENT OF HEALTH & HUMAN SERVICES

Washington, D.C. 20201

STATEMENT OF

HELEN L. SMITS, M.D.

DEPUTY ADMINISTRATOR

HEALTH CARE FINANCING ADMINISTRATION

BEFORE THE

COMMITTEE ON SCIENCE, SPACE AND TECHNOLOGY

UNITED STATES HOUSE OF REPRESENTATIVES

MAY 2, 1994

Mr. Chairman and Members of the Subcommittee:

I welcome this opportunity to discuss the emerging technology of telemedicine and its potential to provide access to quality health care in areas that are traditionally underserved. Although its use is by no means widespread, telemedicine as practiced in existing sites has real potential to improve the availability of the services and advice of medical specialists to primary care practitioners and their patients. The technology is in the process of diffusion, and the real questions are not whether we will be including telemedicine in the mainstream of the nation's health care system, but exactly how it will be used.

In the testimony that follows I will use the term "telemedicine " to refer to two way, interactive video systems over which medical consultation takes place. I am not including the use of telecommunications technology to transport still images, particularly radiologic images, from one site to another. We are quite aware that teleradiology is in common use in many sites, both urban and rural and that Medicare already pays for these services. We are currently exploring the question of quality standards for teleradiology, but do not have questions about the appropriateness of paying for this service when the radiologic image is of sufficient quality.

In the last six months, I have personally visited several active telemedicine demonstration sites. What I saw there made sense from a medical standpoint: telemedicine can be an effective mechanism facilitating the delivery of care. Rural practitioners who regularly seek telemedicine consultation believe their practices are enhanced and their own satisfaction is increased. Consultants providing advice by telemedicine welcome the opportunity to support rural practice and to ensure that patients requiring transfers are appropriately studied and treated at the primary care site. It seems to me that both sides seem to enjoy the consultant/generalist relationship more when telemedicine adds a sense of personal contact.

Telemedicine is a promising means to link rural providers and patients to services not locally available. It also can improve the professional "connectedness" of rural providers and help them keep up with the state of the art of medicine. These features should increase the ability of rural areas to retain rural providers and perhaps even to recruit them. They may also lead to improvement in the appropriateness and quality of care delivered to rural patients.

Another positive aspect of the use of telemedicine is that the television linkages used for consultation can be used to provide continuing education for physicians and nurses as well as degree granting training for a variety of medical personnel. By increasing access to education in rural areas, we can enhance the lives of those who live there and the job satisfaction of practitioners who choose to locate there.

Principles of Coverage for Telemedicine Under Medicare

Although HCFA currently has no explicit national coverage of telemedicine, we do think that the coverage of and payment for telemedical services by Medicare and Medicaid is important for improving access to care and should be explored.

Currently, Medicare covers a physician's services if the physician and patient meet in person in the same room and are "face to face." Under these rules, Medicare cannot cover telemedicine linkages that have the physician on one end and the patient on the other end of the linkage. In order to cover telemedicine consultations, Medicare would have to revise these rules with specific attention as to when and how non face-to-face consultations would be considered to be appropriate care. Since only 2000 total consultations were done in the United States in the past year, we simply do not have the information on which to base such coverage rules.

In the existing sites, telemedicine is facilitated by an efficient organization at the referral site which makes the full spectrum of professional consultation available to the primary care physician twenty-four hours a day and seven days a week. One question which must be answered is whether this type of organization should be required or is an ideal which will be achievable at only a few centers. Clearly not all types of specialties are equally suited to consultation via telemedicine. Patients must also have the choice to make use of a more private means of obtaining consultation when they choose. We also need to evaluate the implications for patient privacy of recording and storing all consultations. Telemedicine raises some complex questions about physician liability and about admitting privileges, the traditional means by which hospitals oversee the quality of care practiced within their walls. We also have concerns about whether direct patient care (doctor to patient) is an effective service and in what circumstances. As telemedicine becomes more widespread, we have concerns, as do many rural physicians, that this technology which ought to support rural practitioners could be used to siphon patients away from rural doctors, thus undercutting one of the principal arguments in favor of the technology. Finally, there are some very experimental types of telemedicine, such as the use of sophisticated computer technology on a non-interactive basis, which deserve evaluation along with the more established face to face systems.

A few of the potential benefits of telemedicine are as follows:

- First, telemedical networks permit the provision of comprehensive, coordinated health care services to rural residents served by the system. These networks use referrals, consultations, and support systems to ensure patient access to a comprehensive set of services.

- Second, telemedical networks can provide the means for rural practitioners to establish ongoing cooperative working relationships with other providers that assure the full range of quality health care services. This infrastructure enables rural practitioners to extend the scope of care they are capable of providing their patients by tapping the expertise of specialists through consultations. It also serves as a means of communication between primary care physicians and specialists, as well as between non-physician primary care practitioners and physicians. For patients who cannot be treated locally, the infrastructure provides referral relationships that include an important feedback loop to the referring rural practitioner. Practitioners using telemedicine argue that networks of care improve practitioner satisfaction as well as patient care.

- Other benefits include increases in the number of patients who can be successfully treated in rural hospitals, and decreases in duplicate testing when patients are transferred out of rural areas for treatment.

On the basis of the information currently available, it appears that telemedicine technology would be most successful if we covered consultations over telemedicine networks that are part of integrated systems of care. Ideally such telemedicine networks would be designed to provide to rural sites a comprehensive range of telecommunication consultations using technology that provides an adequate visual image for communications and diagnosis.

I can envision telemedical networks similar to the active sites at Texas Tech and the Medical College of Georgia that I have recently visited operating in many rural areas. In these networks, the academic health center serves as a hub which makes consultations available on a twenty-four hour basis and has the capacity for follow-up care when necessary. Consultations within the network can also take place between, for example, a primary care practitioner in a remote site and a general surgeon located in a mid-sized town. Primary care physicians, in turn, can use the system to supervise nurse practitioners and physician's assistants.

There is a great deal we need to learn about telemedicine. We encourage those currently using this technology and others who are experimenting with it, both in the public and private sector, to be innovative in bringing efficient and effective care to those in need. At the same time, we need to gather information to help guide those who organize and pay for care--both Medicare and others--as to when this service is best used.

Telemedicine as an Emerging Technology

Even though telemedicine has a history that can be traced back several decades, it is still in many ways in its infancy. While it is clear by now that telemedicine can work technically and medically, we must recognize that we have virtually no experience with this form of delivery of medical services. As federal health programs, such as Medicare and Medicaid, and the private insurance industry examine coverage of telemedical services, we must be cautious that we fully understand both its benefits and its limitations so we can develop appropriate policies regarding when and how we pay for telemedical services and how we safeguard the quality of care.

As HCFA assesses the use of telemedicine, we are keenly aware of our responsibility to assure the quality of care for all who are in the Medicare and Medicaid programs. There must be assurances and specific guidelines in place to provide the same level of quality of care that is present for hands-on consultations and referrals. Use of this technology still does not replace human contact, and we must be sure that the use of telemedicine will not compromise the quality of care for any patient.

Another concern is the whether telemedicine will be accepted and utilized by all providers and by their patients. This type of technology might not be readily supported by physicians or seen as a viable alternative to physically transferring a patient to a tertiary hospital. Particularly once the initial glamour has worn off, patients may be wary of this less private means of communicating. I am sure as use of the technology expands, we will begin to identify circumstances in which its use is less than ideal.

The potential also exists for overuse and inappropriate use of telemedical services. As we develop national policy regarding definitions of the limits of telemedicine, we need to build in appropriate safeguards. We need to construct coverage and payment policies that do not create incentives for practitioners to over-provide services. This is a problem we have experienced with other high technology diagnostic tools such as MRIs and CAT scans. While we welcome the advent of new technology to better serve our beneficiaries, we must be sure that the technology will be used in an appropriate manner that is consistent with medical practice and beneficial to the patient.

81-951 O - 94 - 2

Clearly more assessment and pilot testing must be done to quantify the benefits and potential uses of telemedicine. HCFA is ready to support such efforts and would encourage private industry to participate in expanding telemedicine technology and its clinical applications. I very much hope that we can reach cooperative agreements to exchange information about the use of telemedicine with private insurers so that all payors can have the best possible information base on which to make coverage decisions.

Anticipated Efforts Towards Assessing the Efficacy of Telemedicine

We understand that last year there were fewer than 2,000 telemedical consultations in the U.S. and Canada over a dozen networks. At this time HCFA has very limited data on which to base national policy regarding coverage and payment for telemedical services.

Under these circumstances, we are pursuing answers to questions about telemedicine on a pilot basis. We actively encourage the private insurance industry to also initiate projects to explore the potential applicability of telemedicine in clinical care. A set of pilot projects would enable payors to garner experience while we experiment with a number of approaches. Pilot telemedical networks would provide services on an ongoing basis, and they would furnish payors with information for use in evaluation. Depending on what is learned, we can develop broader coverage and payment rules over time.

I envision that pilot projects will encourage the development of referral relationships between rural providers and specialty care providers and centers. Relationships will be strengthened as the consulting physician receives detailed primary data about the patient in the presence of the referring rural practitioner. By using this available technology and receiving expertise and necessary data from the consulting physician, the referring practitioner can be assisted in diagnosing and recommending treatment for the patient.

Further, we would expect our role to pay only for medical services delivered over telemedicine networks, not that of providing capital funding for starting networks. This is in keeping with our payment role in other areas.

We should point out that grant money for capital costs is available from several sources to fund the start-up costs of initial networks. For example, the Rural Electrification Administration (REA) has allocated $20 million to "encourage, improve and make affordable the use of telecommunications, computer networks and related technology for rural communities to improve access to education and medical and health care". Grants are designed to address some of the following areas: educational and/or medical services which would remain unavailable without advanced technology; technological costs and benefits examining operation, maintenance; evidence of technological and financial need; and potential for "sustainability" when funding terminates.

Additionally, in support of the development of a National Information Infrastructure (NTIA), the National Telecommunications and Information Administration of the Department of Commerce administers the Telecommunications and Information Infrastructure Assistance Program. This program will aid numerous social service providers, including rural health clinics, to obtain connections to telecommunications networks. This year Congress has appropriated $26 million for the program, and the Administration has asked for $100 million in FY 1995 and $150 million for FY 1996. Finally, the House has passed an authorization bill which mandates NTIA to serve as an information clearinghouse for telemedicine applications. With these Congressional directives, NTIA expects to help "jumpstart" the National Information Infrastructure (NII) for a broad range of non-profit social service providers.

Current HHS Support for Telemedicine

The Health Care Financing Administration is already collecting and reviewing some preliminary information on the use of telemedicine. We have contracted with the Center for Health Policy Research (CHPR) in Denver to conduct a review of state-of-the-art telemedicine. The Center is developing a framework to assess the effectiveness of telemedicine.

In Fiscal Year 1994 the HCFA appropriation for research, demonstration, and evaluation activities included $7.25 million over the budget request with $5 million of the increase intended for rural telemedicine grants. This Spring we solicited grant applications for projects that demonstrate the effectiveness of rural telemedicine systems and those that will develop, pilot test, and evaluate payment methodology for telemedicine consultations. We expect to announce grant awards in this area before the end of this month.

The Office of Rural Health Policy in the Public Health Service currently funds a project in West Virginia and has allocated $4 million for approximately 8-10 additional projects. These projects would "demonstrate and collect information on the feasibility, costs, appropriateness, and acceptability of telemedicine consultations for improving access to health services for rural residents and reducing the isolation of rural practitioners." Grant funds may <u>not</u> be used for the costs of purchasing and installing transmission equipment.

Conclusion

In closing, I would like to reiterate that telemedicine has substantial potential to improve access to medical expertise not readily available in underserved areas. While I support the use of telemedicine and believe in its effectiveness, I also recognize that it is an emerging and somewhat untested technology. Because of our limited experience with delivery of telemedical services in the real world, we would like to proceed with caution. However, I can say with confidence, that through the use of pilot projects undertaken by both the Government and private industry, we will be able to learn the best approach to provide effective and efficient health care services for our beneficiaries. HCFA envisions accessible health care being provided through the use of telemedicine and other emerging technologies but it must be based on solid data so that the quality of health care provided is not compromised.

I would be pleased to answer any questions you may have.

Mr. HAYES. Thank you. You have touched upon at the conclusion of your statement something that I wanted to ask earlier. If I were not very interested in this issue and supportive of the concept, we wouldn't be sitting here today trying to build a record for others to read later. But so many things in Government seem to end up getting out of hand by number and hands not knowing which one is where.

Dr. Lindberg remarked that he is aware of and then did an excellent listing, concluded by saying I am sure there are things he doesn't know about. If he doesn't know, I don't know, and if we don't create a structure that allows for the sharing of information that comes to a clearinghouse, we may get ahead of ourselves and have used resources that could have been spent earlier on. Right now where we are going from pioneer programs into your suggestion of having some sites that can serve as pilots, what structure should we suggest and put in place that does know everything, everywhere and can be looked to by each agency as a coordinator of what activities are happening?

Dr. LINDBERG. I think on the side of gathering information, I think a year from now that will be taken care of by NLM. In the past year, Congress provided earmarked funds to us in the area of a health services information center, recognizing that that hadn't been done and it was a new area, not a neglected area, but an area that hadn't been as well organized as traditional biomedical research. So we are well on the way to accomplishing that.

That is not coordinating and doling out resources, that is being aware of all those activities. So I think that that part of it we will take care of. The coordinating and doling out of resources you may have to take care of yourselves.

Mr. HAYES. I wonder, though, through what. We have problems with controversies about earmarking and everything else. Perhaps we could avoid some of our own structural problems if we thought through what the best structure for us to use was.

The second thing I want to ask is what is the best way to create a mechanism that can allow in the future judgment of costs and judgment of potential cost savings as well as judgment of actual cost savings? To be very blunt, a lot of times technology is viewed as the unwilling villain in health care costs and in many instances pointed to by expensive technology, but it is also appropriate to make the conceptual argument that technology is the only way to cut costs down and you can turn it into a VCR example of saying if you have one or two it is expensive but if you are able to network, suddenly individual costs drop; and secondly, what are early care and detection—you mentioned earlier about breast cancer—obviously experience with that if successful would show cost decline, not high cost treatment always at the end.

As a hybrid of my earlier question, what is the best structure to try to impose now to help us learn more about competing costs and to help us try to choose some priorities that would be the best expenditure of money as we make appropriations down the road?

Dr. SMITS. That is one of the questions we want to ask if Congress decides to allow us to establish pilot projects. That would be part of the evaluation. HCFA has its own research evaluating arm and we are working very hard with the Agency for Health Care

Policy and Research to be sure we are coordinated with them and not overlapping. Either we or they ought to undertake a serious look at the cost-effectiveness of these actual projects in place in terms of what it costs the health care system and what benefits it brings to the health care system.

We currently have a contract with the University of Colorado to help us develop a structure to do that.

In terms of cooperation, I think the cooperation inside Health and Human Services has been excellent. We have been working directly with HRSA and with NLM on various parts of this.

It is important to remember that to a great extent, these systems will work well and be affordable in very small towns if they do more than telemedicine. They can also involve distant learning plans even at the elementary school level. The project I saw in Texas, kept their lines busy almost full-time doing educational programs of various types, continuing education for the practitioners on the line—it is a wonderful way that you can train individuals in small towns, for technically—for jobs that require technical training, such as licensed practical nursing courses.

There is also a lot of exciting interaction we can do. So you can't hold it too close inside health because it will work best if cooperative with the rest of the information infrastructure. I understand that Commerce currently within the information infrastructure is where that coordination is going on relative to telemedicine. There also are coordinating committees established by the Administration for the NII work that are specific to health care.

Mr. HAYES. Thank you. Ms. Morella.

Mrs. MORELLA. I appreciated the testimony that both of you presented. In listening to the possibilities, when you mentioned, Dr. Lindberg, mental health, I was thinking that we could eventually perhaps get rid of the metal detectors which screen people as they go into the Capitol building and put mental detectors. Many applications.

Is the Federal Government leading the way in the attempt? You both have mentioned many of the Federal agencies involved, albeit Commerce and Energy and all the others—what is the role at this point of the private sector?

Is it the Federal Government that is the engine steering this?

Dr. LINDBERG. I think inevitably the Federal Government has to lead the way in terms of networking because there is no other way it can happen. It is not an economical proposition to be in the business of gigabit transportivity. That is not a way to make money. That is why we have gigabit test bed sites. Only one of the six is a medical site. That is at Chapel Hill.

But I have talked with the HPCC side with the companies, in that case it would be Bell Atlantic and they are producing products that come out of the gigabit test beds in spite of the fact they can't yet sell million bit transmission to individuals. The Government is leading the way and doing a good job.

On the application side, I think that inventiveness is going to come from the universities and the hospitals and medical schools and bioengineers and people who usually do that and the Government role is through peer review and support through the grant mechanism. I think the intellectual leadership will come from individuals as it always has.

Dr. SMITS. I think that given who is in the audience, it is important to stress how indebted we are to the individuals, particularly often in State settings in universities who have helped set these networks up and have been committed to developing them. The Government role, it seems to me, there are some issues and standard setting and by being sure that the roads are there and that the vehicles can get around the roads. But this is a very exciting private sector development with, I think, a very positive collaboration.

They didn't do it without us and we didn't do it without them. I would hate to sit here and look Jay Sanders in the eye and say the Federal Government gets all the credit.

Mrs. MORELLA. Is there a branch within the executive agency that tries to coordinate? It seems like we have mentioned a lot of different agencies. But is there something coordinating?

Dr. LINDBERG. Sure. OSTP. The high performance computer program involves 10 agencies, and it reports to the President's science advisor, Jack Gibbons. I think in the area of these big systems, be it the computer side or the communications side or Internet, the reason that the 10 agency program was put together was because none could do it alone. They didn't have the resources. They had the needs and not the ability and they didn't have the application side, which may be one of the reasons that biomedicine has been prominent.

I think it was inevitable that the agencies had to pool their problems and resources and NLM manages it.

Mrs. MORELLA. Let me ask you about your high performance computing and communications leadership, you had a significant increase in your budget. Are there additional responsibilities that you are taking over now for that and how does that tie into the telemedicine?

Dr. LINDBERG. Pretty close really, because in the legislation the Congress is currently considering, S. 4 and H.R. 1757, there is another bill, H. 20 that is involved but basically the National Information Infrastructure and Applications Act.

In that, four application areas are singled out: health care, education and lifelong learning, digital libraries and advanced manufacturing, to which the House added public access to Government information. Those are the application areas.

Health is very prominent in that. In the legislation still under consideration, there were six elements of the health care provisions and when we did this broad agency announcement that I spoke of, we essentially used word-for-word, the six health care provisions, the first one of which was a test bed network. That is what we are using our money to fund.

We think we have some empirical evidence on a statewide regional basis of how well it is going to work. The second was collaborative arrangements for treating patients at a distance. Again, that technology is important, but the arrangements amongst the people in the organizations are even more important and difficult.

The third element is, let's say, advanced image processing and virtual reality which gives you feedback and control of examinations.

The fourth area is a very big area at the moment, very underfunded and that is the computer-based record. That is almost the Holy Grail. Without that, it will be hard to do this optimally. In any event, NLM's role was to make that announcement and evaluate the applications, about 140 in number from 31 States. It was a very popular program. We couldn't fund more than 8 or 9 percent of very good applications.

Mrs. MORELLA. That is very interesting. We talk about cost as an important factor that we have got to peruse and pursue further, and as we talk about health care costs, many people have said technology is the major villain, and I have a quote from Dr. Koop in a Los Angeles Times article the other day, and he said that telemedicine is necessary to have the kind of health reform that the administration has planned.

I am wondering if you would like to comment on whether you agree with Dr. Koop's assessment and also what we do with regard to the concept of is technology raising health care costs?

Dr. SMITS. I think what Dr. Koop means by that is what I mentioned, that the sense of isolation in the very remote rural practitioners is acute and painful and that you are not going to keep good physicians in Alpine, Texas or good nurse practitioners at the Texas-Mexican border unless you can assure them that they have continued access to modern medicine. Some of that is telemedicine, face-to-face televised consultations so the patient without a car isn't asked to drive 300 miles; some of it is Internet, access to library work, a whole lot of general access to information. It changes the way people feel about practicing in very remote areas and coverage isn't enough. Universal coverage won't change that isolation. Availability of support for those practitioners will. It will help attract and it will help retain people.

Mrs. MORELLA. How do you see the administration's health reform plan utilizing telemedicine, if medicare and medicaid is not reimbursing?

Dr. SMITS. As I have indicated—this is a personal statement—if I were running a qualified health plan that included a rural area, I would be very eager to include telemedicine. The fact that Medicare can't write fee-for-service rules yet doesn't mean that it is inappropriate for use in a controlled managed care setting. We want to move ahead with collecting the information so that we can write coverage rules.

In that sense—in fact, I believe that our authorization to do so in pilot sites will probably come with whatever reform bill comes forward to Congress. I think they are very closely tied. I have talked to people at the sites that now exist.

I think it would be unfortunate if this technology, like some others, got over-used too soon. That is, it is possible to imagine a misuse or inappropriate use of this technology, and we need to know enough to protect ourselves from that and to define what is appropriate use before it comes into universal coverage.

Mrs. MORELLA. I guess you would agree, Dr. Lindberg, that it would take awhile to develop the total kind of credibility in the minds of people who would be the users? You have to educate people?

Dr. LINDBERG. I do believe that in medicine the proper diagnosis and the proper long-range treatment plan is in the long run the most inexpensive way to go. I have been involved in experiments now for almost 20 years in rheumatology in which we deploy an expert system, computer-based expert system to help with diagnosis and management decisions.

I was on the President's Commission on Arthritis and Musculoskeletal Disease in 1976. I learned in that session that only 2 to 3 percent of the people in the United States who have those diseases ever see an expert rheumatologist even once, even for diagnosis and a long-range plan. So that most of the treatment, therefore, is done by others, by general practitioners, who may be specialists but not in their field.

We also are convinced that the specialist does a better and cheaper job and a job less fraught with complications. So we tried to package that wisdom and amplify the abilities of the expert. We are just completing field trials in two States now to see how well that works out. Where there is a difficulty is not in the logic of the program. We make the right diagnosis—we are not certain that the non-specialist is able or does make the accurate observation to feed into the program. So we may end up wishing that we had the interactive TV as a second phase.

Mrs. MORELLA. So it becomes more important even since health care reform stresses primary care. If you are stressing primary care, you need to have experts that are going to get further kinds of attention by virtue of telemedicine. You are going to use them more often. It is true, I guess as we go on with the other panels we will learn more about what to do with licensure and confidentiality and piracy and privacy and tort reform.

I thank both of you for your leadership. Dr. Lindberg, it is always a pleasure to hear you and what you are doing. Thank you, Dr. Smits.

Mr. HAYES. I have a related question. You used Alpine, Texas as an example. I wonder if you have been to Alpine, Texas?

Dr. SMITS. No, I would love to go. I have been to Lubbock, and I have talked to the two practitioners at Alpine.

Mr. HAYES. It is a two hour drive after you land at the airport at Lubbock, and you will drive through ranches that are bigger than Ms. Morella's district. There is not a hotel there. There is a four-room boarding house. I have been there, and will you please, after you visit, tell Dan Rather it is not a junket because it is in the middle of nowhere.

Dr. SMITS. I am glad to hear there is a boarding house. I would like to go. I am a great admirer of the two family practitioners who practice there. I have seen a lot of their consults on the videos. I think they are great guys.

Dr. LINDBERG. Lubbock itself is 500 miles from anywhere.

Dr. SMITS. But the barbecue is excellent. Maybe that is what made it a junket.

Mr. HAYES. Thank you both.

The subcommittee is pleased to recognize Dr. Jay Sanders, who is the director of the Telemedicine Center and Professor of Medicine at the Medical College of Georgia, and I hope next Dr. Eric Tangalos, Associate Professor of Medicine at the Mayo Clinic, and

Dr. Edward Gomez, Lieutenant Colonel, U.S. Army, who is the chief of, it says here, to correct my previous text, of Peripheral Vascular Surgery at Walter Reed.

I want to tell you, Colonel, that peripheral vascular surgery struck me, as a layman, as someone whose hand-eye coordination is not the best. Maybe you can explain that to us at some point in your statement. Thank all of you.

We will begin with Dr. Sanders, if you would.

STATEMENT OF DR. JAY H. SANDERS, M.D., DIRECTOR, TELEMEDICINE CENTER, MEDICAL COLLEGE OF GEORGIA, AUGUSTA, GA

Dr. JAY SANDERS. It is a pleasure for me to be here. What I thought I would do is give you an overview of the statewide telemedicine initiative that presently exists at the Medical College of Georgia. With reference to implementation of issues, I have handed out a write-up which will address the majority of those issues, and I would be happy to deal with them in more detail during the question and answer period of time.

In November of 1991, under the leadership and commitment of the governor of the State of Georgia, Governor Bill Miller and the President of the Medical College at Georgia, a partnership amongst the State government, private industry, particularly Southern Bell and Georgia Power and Light, the Medical College of Georgia, and the community, began a State-wide telemedicine initiative.

That began with a single hookup between the Medical College of Georgia and a small community hospital 130 miles southwest of Augusta, Georgia. That was November of 1991. By September of this year, there will be 60 telemedicine facilities throughout the State, and in essence from a functional standpoint, a patient any place in the State of Georgia will be able to be seen and examined by a physician any place in the State of Georgia.

The system is designed based upon the end user's needs and not upon the technologist's desires. The system is open. It is modular, it is back adaptable to improvements in the technology. I want to underline at this point in time that the technology is totally off-the-shelf technology, and I would not define it as high technology.

It is, in fact, inexpensive technology. It is easy to use and we have found that within a 15 to 20 minute period of time for physicians at both sites of the system, they are able to learn the entire use of the system.

The system is totally interactive, real time, and is remotely controlled from both ends so physicians at both sites have the opportunity to manipulate the cameras and see each other in whatever fashion they would like.

To date, since November of 1991, the data that we have accumulated has demonstrated that 85 percent of the patients who previously had to be transferred out of the rural community to a secondary or tertiary care center are now kept in that rural community, in essence, maintaining the revenue stream within the rural community, in that rural community hospital with that rural community physician.

The system is only activated by the rural-based physician, so there is not any competitive mode that exists here. This is something that is developed to be complementary to and to sustain both the professional and the economic lifeblood of the rural community as well as the rural-based physician.

If I could show some slides, I would like to give you an idea of the system. The system was developed to meet these particular needs. We needed to go out to the rural communities to define what the problems were in terms of rural health care, and what we quickly identified was that the lack of specialty care necessitated that the patient who required a cardiologist or neurologist would quickly have to be discharged from that rural hospital.

That discharge immediately impacted on the bed census of the hospital which in essence undermined the fiscal stability of that rural hospital. But we found out something even more significant, and that is that because in most rural communities the rural hospital represents the major employer, we were not only impacting on the fiscal stability of the hospital; we were impacting on the socioeconomic fabric of that community.

The issue of professional isolation was clearly identified by Dr. Smits. What happens in medical school, all medical students, all physicians are trained in major academic medical centers where they become addicted to all of their subspecialty colleagues and all the types of high technology.

Then we cut that educational umbilical cord and the individual ends up in the real world. That type of professional isolation is very clear, but the other part of the professional isolation was the professional isolation on the part of people like myself.

I have spent my entire professional career in academic medicine as a teacher, and yet the reality is that if I had to go out tomorrow to set up a practice in a rural community, I would not have the slightest idea how to do that, and yet I am the one training that individual.

So what we wanted to do was to ensure that there was also—that we also got rid of the professional isolation in the academic community as to what the real world of medicine was like.

We identified very quickly that there was significant discontinuity of care between the patient and his or her physician when that transfer occurred, and certainly between the patient and his or her relative. All of that impacted on the quality of care.

We also noted that continuing medical education in the rural communities was totally ineffective. It was occurring at the wrong time, at the wrong place, by the wrong individuals. This rural-based physician needed an answer to a question immediately at the time that they had a question about their patient. They couldn't wait for three to six months to go off to a major medical center to sit in a lecture hall and to be lectured to by a lecturer who was talking about what his or her interests were, not really what the particular interests and needs of that primary care physician was.

And one of the striking things we noted was that if we put a patient in a rural hospital bed in Georgia, the per average day cost was $800 a day. The minute we transferred that patient to the Medical College of Georgia because they may have had to have seen a cardiologist or neurologist, the per average day cost was $1,300 a day.

The simple transfer from one bed in a rural site to a bed in an urban community was an increase of $500 a day and that did not include the cost of transportation, it did not include the cost of loss of productivity, and it certainly did not include the cost of increased severity of illness, because if I wait until tomorrow to treat your infection rather than initiating antibiotic therapy today, the likelihood is that tomorrow your disease process was going to be more severe.

So we developed this type of interactive telemedicine system, and as the previous speakers have said, this is just one end of the pendulum. This is not the totality of telemedicine. The telephone is the beginning of a telemedicine consultation. This is a real time, interactive, audio visual link, and here we have a cardiologist at the Medical College of Georgia who is examining the patient 130 miles away utilizing an electronic stethoscope.

The nice thing, as Dr. Smits mentioned, here from our standpoint is the fact that we see something different than we usually see in the traditional consultative patient interaction, and that is that the referring physician at Dodge County Hospital, the primary care physician, has chosen to stay in the room with her patient at the time that the consultation is occurring.

Now, the system in no way dictates the need for that specialist, that primary care physician to do that, and in studies that we did in the 1970s under a National Science Foundation grant, we identified the fact that simply having a nurse practitioner at the remote site allows the quality of care to be totally maintained.

But what is nice about this setting is that while the cardiologist is listening to this patient's heart and lung sounds, the primary care physician is also listening to those heart and lung sounds and this specialist can say, did you notice how that murmur intensified when we sat that patient up? That is classically seen in floppy mitral valve.

This physician gets immediate on-line continuing medical education based upon what her question is, not based upon what the interests of the cardiologist might be.

In fact, as I will shortly show you, this physician, this physician here at the Medical College of Georgia, can do a total examination of this patient at the remote site by looking in that patient's retina, ears, nose and throat, listening to the heart and lung sounds.

He can review the chest x-ray, electrocardiogram or cardiac ultrasound, and we asked both the patient and the consulting physician to sign a single-page form, and we have never had a patient or physician refuse, and that allows us to capture the entire examination.

So that when this patient comes back three weeks from now and I want to compare his heart and lung sounds with what it sounded like three weeks previously, I can bring back that entire cardiopulmonary examination.

Here is the referring physician at the remote site with her patient interacting with the specialist back at the medical center.

Now, as I mentioned, the system is modular and has open architecture. There are 15 major components to the system. They are all off the shelf, but when the half life of one of these components is up, we don't have to throw the entire system away. The system is totally compatible with the new technology. We just unplug the old component.

This is a standard VCR where we captured part of the consultation. We use this for risk management, quality assurance, as well as this becomes our teaching file. These are the controls for our electronic stethoscope which allow us to do things with our electronic stethoscope that the cardiologist, in fact, cannot do at the bedside in your room.

And here we have a standard fax machine which allows us, in a situation in which the physician may not be computer literate, for her to write or dictate the note and it is immediately faxed out to the remote site. In addition, what we do is we have an on-line database so that if I have just seen a patient as a consultant who has floppy mitral valve, and I want that physician who has referred the patient to know that that patient needs to be on antibiotic prophylaxis prior to any type of surgical procedure, I have not only examined the patient with that referring physician, I have not only discussed the patient with her, but I have written a note, and now I will provide an up-to-date medical reference for that physician at the remote site and that gets immediately incorporated into the patient's chart.

Now, this is a hand-held, off-the-shelf device called a microscopical camera. It is very similar to the camera that surgeons now use to do laparoscopic surgery. This is a camera that is placed in your abdomen during laparoscopic surgery and in fact the doctor is not looking at you any longer when he is doing the operation. He is actually looking at a TV screen at the foot—at the head of the operating table, and he is watching what his hands are doing in your abdomen by looking at that TV monitor.

Well, what we found out very early on is that we could take this camera with some very simple adapters on the end of that camera, such as this, and in effect attach that camera to any standard medical scope. Here is the standard ENT, ear, nose and throat otoscope and here is the ophthalmoscope.

We take the otoscope to look in your ears, nose and throat with the adapter hooked onto the camera, and now we can allow our primary care physician at the remote site to look in his patient's ear at the time that our ear, nose and throat specialist is looking at the patient's ear 130 miles away, and I should mention that that patient can be 13,000 miles away.

We are using digital signaling and it adapts to any type of communication mode that you have. In fact, our chairman of ENT has stated that he can actually see the middle ear better over this digital signal because we can enhance this picture in a way that he cannot do if that patient were in his office.

But in addition to the otoscope and ophthalmoscope, we can hook this to any scope, a gastroscope, colonoscope, bronchioscope, arthroscope, cystoscope and we can also transmit the pathologist. With the microscopical camera here screwed onto the teaching head of the microscope, we can get second and primary decisions made by a pathologist back at the medical center.

In essence with this simple off-the-shelf camera, we can create an electronic umbilical cord between all of the sub-specialty expertise that exists at the major medical centers with all of the community hospitals.

It became apparent to us with use of the system that, in fact, a single bay station at the Medical College of Georgia can network with multiple remote sites and multiple remote health care markets.

We have identified up to this point in time, this is preliminary data, we are doing a much more comprehensive evaluation at the present time as the program is being expanded, that we have provided immediate access to care for the patient, we have decreased professional isolation for the physicians at both ends, both at the rural site and the academic community. We have enhanced continuing medical education and we have enhanced continuity of care.

I just want to underline the fact that 85 percent of the patients who previously had to be transferred out of that rural community are now kept in the rural community.

Therefore, we have increased the revenue stream for that remote hospital and we have kept the economy of that community stabilized. We have increased the revenue of that primary health care provider, and remember the differential between the $800 a day bed and the $1,300 a day bed.

This is the present system at the Medical College of Georgia. We are connected to rural hospitals, freestanding ambulatory health care facilities, a public health facility and correctional institutions.

Under a Phase 1 study, which will be—expansion which will be completed within the next 45 days, we are adding four secondary hubs in Gainesville, Columbus, Albany and Waycross. From each of those secondary hubs, there will be satellite facilities spoking out to underserved sites.

And by September of this year, we will be adding an additional six hub facilities, another tertiary care center similar to MCG at Emory, and from each of the additional hubs, a total of nine secondary hubs and two tertiary hubs, there will be three to four satellites.

In essence, by the end of September of 1994, there will be 60 sites throughout the State and in fact, because of the communication infrastructure that has been developed in the State of Georgia, a patient any place in the State, let me give you an example, parents down here in Bainbridge, Georgia which may just have had a child with cystic fibrosis and they need to see a geneticist and their child needs to see a pediatric pulmonary specialist who knows about DNAs, that child and those parents in Bainbridge, Georgia will first access their secondary hub in Thomasville. However, if the expertise, in terms of a geneticist and pediatric pulmonary specialist does not exist in Thomasville, those parents and that patient in Bainbridge can be seen by any physician throughout the State.

Now, a great New Yorker slide that I like to use to underline two things that we are presently working on, number one is the one thing we can't do at the present time over our telemedicine system is literally reach out and touch our patient, and with Georgia Tech, we are working on an electronic hand to be able to transmit the full sensation that your hand can provide.

But more importantly in this slide is something that we are really excited about, and that is, once we have our State-wide network, we really need to go where health care needs to be provided, and we need to keep a patient from becoming a patient in the first place, and we need to keep people out of our emergency department, and the best way for us to do that is to begin to take the entire functionality that I just showed you between a major medical center and a rural hospital and literally, in fact, bring it into your living room, and now working with the cable industry and the telephone industry in the State of Georgia, we will be identifying 25 homes in the greater Augusta area.

In fact, the cable that now brings you your HBO and Cinemax into your home can very easily technologically, with some simple reverse amplifiers, be made totally interactive and you will turn on not your Home Shopping Channel, but your Home Medical Channel, and you will, in fact, be able to see and talk to your physician in his office or at the hospital.

We will get T–1 band width out of that cable that you now have, with a camcorder camera on top of your TV monitor, and what we are now calling a smart box, which will contain an electronic stethoscope, an EKG, a pulse oximeter to take blood oxygen levels, a Doppler blood pressure and pulse cuff, and some other pulmonary function devices, we will, in fact, be able to see our patients at home and identify long before their illness becomes so severe that they need to be in the hospital emergency room; we will be able to interact with them and initiate therapy at a much less severe stage of their illness so that hopefully we will be able to keep them out of the emergency department.

We are calling this project our Back to the Future project. We are replacing the black bag house call with the electronic house call.

And my favorite Gary Larsen cartoon to sum up, a heard of buffalo, all stampeding in the same direction and one buffalo saying to another, if we all knew where we were going—as if we all knew where we were going. That is the telemedicine program at the Medical College of Georgia.

[The prepared statement of Jay H. Sanders, M.D. follows:]

TELEMEDICINE

CHALLENGES TO IMPLEMENTATION

Presented to the Subcommittee on Investigations
and Oversight
Washington D.C.
May 2, 1994

Jay H. Sanders
Professor of Medicine
Director, Telemedicine Center
Eminent Scholar of Telemedicine
Medical College of Georgia

Jonathan S. Sanders, Esq.

It is ironic that despite dramatic advances in our ability to care for patients, our ability to translate that knowledge into an accessible, affordable health care system remains an elusive goal. As a result, millions of people have been unable to obtain even the most basic of health care needs. Socio-economic and geographical barriers for patients, compounded by educational isolation for physicians, underline the problems. Providing a patient health care where and when it is needed with an assurance of quality and an economy of cost clearly must be the objective of any health care delivery system. Since the present system does not satisfy these criteria, alternatives are needed. Telemedicine has been proposed as one of those alternatives. However, if telemedicine is to play a significant role, a number of implementation and operational issues will need to be addressed.

Licensure

It is anticipated that, based on the present individual state licensure system, a physician utilizing telemedicine to provide consultative services to a patient would have to be licensed in every state that the patient resided. Given the often burdensome process involved in obtaining state licensure it is unlikely that many physicians will pursue that avenue and, thus, potentially significantly limit the networking capability that this telecommunication system affords.

A number of potential solutions are proposed:

(1) individual state licensure for telemedicine should be converted to a national licensure similar to the military health care system. In fact, since physicians are required to take national examinations for licensure and certification it seems illogical to have a system of individual state licensure

in the first place. Perhaps, in order to assess the impact of such a change, a "national" license could be provided to those physicians who provide telemedicine consultations to patient populations that have been defined as "underserved";
(2) in the instance of a specialty consultation requested by the primary care physician, the referring physician retains responsibility for the care of that patient, and, therefore any "care" provided over telemedicine by the consulting physician in another state could be viewed as recommendations only;
(3) perhaps the most logical way to deal with state licensure requirements is to determine that the patient is, in fact, being "electronically transported" to the physician rather than the physician being transported to the patient.

Another licensure issue that surfaces when considering telemedicine consultations across state lines is whether the Federal Trade Commission would view this as interstate commerce.

Credentialing

Although issues similar to the licensing debate can be raised with reference to credentialing, it would appear that an opinion provided by the Joint Commission on Accreditation of Healthcare Organizations for the Medical College of Georgia telemedicine system could be uniformly applicable. The JCAHO determined that a physician at MCG who provided a telemedicine consultation of a patient at Dodge County Hospital (a rural hospital 130 miles distant from MCG) would not have to be credentialed at that rural hospital as long as any orders written in the patient's chart were by the referring physician at Dodge County Hospital. The consulting physician is not considered the physician responsible for the care of the patient.

Liability/Malpractice

Malpractice liability may prove to be one of the most vexing problems and could impede the general application of telemedicine. Obviously, any analysis of "what might be" will only gain validity from the outcome of precedent setting cases.

Although, to date, we have no evidence of any malpractice activity having been generated by past and present telemedicine initiatives, one can anticipate that as reimbursement becomes a reality, and as medical centers with "deep pockets" who become networked with remote sites are viewed in an "agency" relationship, more attention will be paid to this area by the legal profession. It also should be recognized that those telemedicine systems that utilize digital compression technology to transmit images will have a very special type of liability exposure, namely, that the "data" being reviewed by the consulting physician is not complete! Finally, the inability, at present, for telemedicine systems to allow for actual "hands on" examination of the patient will serve to foster the perception that a telemedicine consultation is incomplete or inadequate.

Clearly, a preventative approach to liability is the best defense. It must be stressed to the physician that if the visual/audio links do not provide adequate information transfer to allow for appropriate diagnostic interpretation none should be made. Videotaping of the entire consultative exchange will provide excellent record keeping and avoid the common pitfall of lack of documentation. Telemedicine systems that provide access to up-to-date references as well as the expanding library of "practice guidelines" now being introduced by the specialty societies will help to address the issue of whether the care provided by the physician satisfied community standards. Perhaps the doctrine of "sovereign immunity" could be applied to those physicians/medical centers that offer telemedicine consultations to the underserved.

Confidentiality

The transmission of personal and sensitive medical information over communication lines clearly lends itself to electronic intrusion and exposure. Encrypting algorithms will need to be introduced but it is naive to think that even the most sophisticated code could not be broken. Once again legal precedent will determine the standard, but it is likely that if "reasonable and customary" efforts are taken to maintain the security of records this issue will not be difficult to resolve. In fact, if one examines the fairly open access to patient records that prevails in our existing system it can be expected that the electronic transfer of medical information may have more security.

Recordkeeping

As has been noted, videotaping will allow for more accurate, as well as, expanded capture of medical information. However, medical records will exist at both ends of the communication link, thus raising the question as to which record reflects the legal one. How are we going to "edit" the vast amount of information retrieved, and will deletion of "unimportant" components of the patient's history and physical examination be considered record tampering?

Technology - Design/Operation/Maintenance

Today any technology-based system needs to share the following characteristics: (1) adaptability to change; (2) ease of operation, and (3) minimal maintenance requirements.

Changes in communication technology and information processing and management are occurring at a more rapid pace than even the most optimistic predictions. It is essential, therefore, that any multicomponent telemedicine system have an open architecture and modular design that can adapt to upgrades with component replacement rather than system extinction. Technical expertise should be a prerequisite only for the integrator of the system not the people using it. System controls must be user-friendly and incorporated into a single control panel. Every effort should be made to convert the present configuration, in which a separate telemedicine consultative room is utilized, to a more flexible desktop multi-media platform that is accessible to the physician in his/her office. Portability must also be a prerequisite to allow for the deployment of transportable telemedicine units that can service multiple remote facilities on an "as needed basis." System maintenance needs to be the simplest task of all - modularity of system components, telephone dial-up maintenance assessment algorithms, and "strategic" redundancy need to be incorporated into the system design. Most importantly, the design of the system must be dictated by the needs of the end-users not those of the system architect. Functionality must control structure and the technology should have a transparent interface between users.

Operational personnel requirements are minimal. A single FTE at each site can manage system operation, scheduling of the consultations and preventative maintenance responsibilities. If the base station system is situated in proximity to the emergency department, telemedicine consultations can be made available to the remote rural hospital on a 24-hour per day basis.

Technological Compatibility

It is imperative that equipment manufacturers strive for competitive similarities rather than proprietary constructs. Systems that can't "speak" the same language will never integrate with each other, and, thus, will paralyze network development. Witness the minimal use of facsimile machines prior to the introduction of a common language and the explosion in sales when a common alphabet was introduced.

Value/Economics

Telemedicine must be identified as a value added service to maintain its viability, and central to that objective, is that it be cost effective. Preliminary data from the MCG telemedicine system demonstrates that 81% of the patients who are seen over telemedicine have not required transfer to a secondary or tertiary care center. Given an average cost differential of $500 per day between the rural hospital bed ($800) and that at the Medical College of Georgia ($1300), even a 25% decrease in transfers would be a significant cost savings. Add to that the savings in transportation costs, increased productivity, and the decreased hospitalization days resulting from treating a patient at an earlier stage in their disease process, and it is apparent that the potential savings are significant. Consider also that the health care revenue generated is staying at the rural site thus enhancing not only the fiscal stability of that hospital but also the socio-economic fabric of that community. Finally, in contrast to most new medical technology, telemedicine systems do not require major capital investments, and the cost of individual components continue to fall as the technology improves. Despite the relatively low cost, however, it is recommended that rural health care facilities, in order to conserve cash flow, lease the system over a three to five year time frame allowing the revenue generated by the anticipated increase in bed census and ambulatory activity to offset the leasing costs. (The leasing contract should provide for component upgrades so that the system always remains at the cutting edge.) Assuming that the average cost of a satellite site if purchased outright is about $160,000, it should be noted that an increase of a single patient to the average per day bed census represents a net cash flow of $150,000/year to the hospital. However, despite the reduced capital expenditure many rural hospitals will still not have the needed start-up funding. If that is the case, then it is recommended that government (local, state and/or federal) provide a loan to "pump prime" these facilities. As revenue is generated the rural hospital will then be able to assume the monthly leasing costs as well as payback the start-up loan.

Educational Value

Perhaps one of the most important applications of telemedicine that will significantly foster its implementation is its capacity to alter the state of professional isolation that now exists for the rural based physician. Telemedicine addresses each of the necessary characteristics of an effective CME experience namely that the information provided is (1) timely, (2) pertinent to the issue, (3) convenient to obtain, (4) repetitive and (5) up-to-date. By providing immediate access to colleagues at the medical center, telemedicine creates an "electronic umbilical cord" between the two facilities, and allows for a real-time interactive educational experience for the referring physician. As importantly, it helps the academic based consultant to be more aware of, and sensitive to, the needs of the rural-based physician. An added fringe benefit is that, depending on the nature, format and comprehensiveness of the consultative interchange, it is possible to grant category I CME credits to the rural-based physician. The significance of obtaining these credits is underlined by the fact that in many states relicensure is dependent on having accumulated these credits and without this on-site opportunity afforded by telemedicine the process is both inconvenient and expensive.

Communication Costs

Telemedicine systems can interface with a variety of communication modalities (copper wire telephone lines, fiberoptic cable, microwave and satellite) thereby providing maximum flexibility for interconnectivity between sites. One problem with the use of telephone lines, however, is the complex rate structure that exists between LANs that create unrealistic communication costs. Although the introduction of ATM switching and fiberoptic cable will dramatically reduce per use cost, until those technologies are more generally available lower transmission costs for telemedicine will need to be structured to make it economically feasible for rural hospitals to participate.

Motivation for Providers and Patients

It is clear that a number of factors need to be in operation for both physician and patients to use the system, but, perhaps the most fundamental, is for the "users" to recognize a simple paradigm shift. One of the interesting aspects of telemedicine is the perception on the part of both physician and patient that this technology is futuristic. In fact, it incorporates all "off-the-shelf" technology. The telecommunications, cameras, remote control optics and examination devices are utilized on a day-to-day basis by each of us simply in different settings. With the same technology that allows us to watch a news anchor interact in real time with his/her correspondent in a distant part of the globe, or view through the use of a telephoto close-up lens, a distant landscape in intimate detail, so too can we examine a patient at a remote site.

For the rural based physician other operational motivating issues require that: (1) the time involved in a telemedicine consultation must integrate into his/her daily schedule and, if the physician can not participate in the consultation, a nurse at the remote end would suffice to allow for an effective examination by the consulting physician; (2) the consultation be reimbursable; (3) the consultation not be competitive; (4) continuity of care, by avoiding unnecessary referrals to secondary or tertiary care centers, be increased; (5) the physician's revenue stream be enhanced; (6) the consultation functions as an effective educational experience; (7) the system be easy to use; and (8) most importantly, it be perceived by that physician's patient as an effective consultative exchange.

Many of the critical factors outlined for the rural based physician hold true for the consulting physician. Economy of time, ease of use and a method for reimbursement are obvious needs. Perhaps the most difficult hurdle that telemedicine needs to clear is to satisfy the technical requirements of the consulting physician. To achieve this it is important that the system architect understands those needs prior to designing the system. Resolution capabilities are critical for the radiologist/pathologist: technological simplicity and user friendliness characterize the need of the mental health care professional, and audio quality of the electronic stethoscope and real time transmission of echocardiograms identify the desire of the cardiologist. Experience from previous telemedicine initiatives have taught us to anticipate that each specialist will come with a different expectation of the systems capability. This needs to be addressed and understood by those who endorse the introduction of telemedicine into the healthcare delivery system.

The ultimate test of the value of telemedicine will be dependent on how the patient perceives and adapts to it. If the patient feels the technology makes the consultation too impersonal; if the telemedicine consultation costs more and is not covered by insurance, and if the patient wants to have the physician literally at their side, telemedicine will not be an acceptable delivery system. In the same manner that there is a learning curve for the physician, we can anticipate a similar situation for the patient. A system that is designed to allow direct eye-to-eye contact, that is easy to use, and that gives the patient the ability to control the interview camera has been shown in previous telemedicine systems to be very "patient friendly." In fact, the patient has perceived himself or herself as being treated in a very special way. In the final analysis it will be the human component at each end of the system - not the technology - that will determine whether it is successful or not. Once again the design of the system must be determined by the needs of the people who use it!

Other Uses

It should be recognized that the telecommunication link between sites can be used for multiple purposes, including administrative meetings, nursing and other allied health educational or direct patient care activities. Telemedicine sites could also be integrated into a state's distance learning initiative so that preventative health care programs as well as acute episodic care intervention can be introduced to the classroom.

Continuous Quality Improvement - CQI

As with any component of the health care system, new or old, there must be regular oversight evaluation to ensure that the objectives for which it was introduced are continuing to be met. Economic viability, quality care, accessible service, appropriate utilization and educational strengths will need to be regularly verified in order to justify the continued operational status of the system.

Conclusion

This paper has attempted to sketch a picture of some of the issues related to the implementation of telemedicine. Whatever new directions or programs we eventually initiate to impact the problems in our health care delivery system it must be coupled with a commitment to analyze and critique them. Despite the feeling that changes need to be made rapidly, solutions cannot come overnight. While tradition can not justify maintaining the present inequities, a new idea can not simply be equated with a proven solution. New programs must be developed to provide the flexibility to accommodate to a wide variety of practice situations and a built-in mechanism to respond to changes in program objectives.

The true measure of the performance of any new system will be whether it effects an improvement in the health of the people it serves. Finally to those of us who believe that telemedicine is a solution close at hand and will require only simple changes we had best heed the words of the philosopher John Gardner. "Social change is a learning process for all concerned. It always requires reeducation of large numbers of people to accept new objectives, new values, new procedures. It can not go forward without the breaking down of long established ways of doing and thinking. This is true whether the problem is one of civil rights, the reform of local government, educational improvement, or urban renewal. Most human institutions are designed to resist such learning rather than facilitate it."

Bibliography

Bashshur RL, Armstrong PA, Youssef ZI. Telemedicine: Explorations in the Use of Telecommunications in Health Care; Charles C. Thomas, Publisher, Springfield, Illinois, USA, 1975.

Sanders JH. The General Internist; Archives of Internal Medicine, September 9, 1977;137:1274-76.

Sanders JH, Tedesco FJ. Telemedicine: Bringing Medical Care to Isolated Communities; Journal of the Medical Association of Georgia, May 1993;82:237-41.

Sanders JH, Sasmor L. Telecommunications in health care delivery. Proceedings of the First Symposium on Research Applied to National Needs (RANN), National Science Foundation, 1973:167-69.

Sanders JH. Increasing productivity through telecommunications. Proceedings of the NSF Symposium on Research Applied to National Needs (RANN-2). November 1976:95.

Preston J, Brown FW, Hartley B. Using Telemedicine to Improve Health Care in Distant Areas; Hospital and Community Psychiatry, January 1993:43:1:25-31.

Gardner JW. Problem Solving; No Easy Victories, Harper and Row, New York, 1968; Chapter 5:27-28.

TELEMEDICINE: Bringing Medical Care to Isolated Communities

Jay H. Sanders, MD, Francis J. Tedesco, MD

Using an interactive voice and color video telecommunication system integrated with biomedical telemetry, physicians at a medical hub can examine and treat patients at multiple satellite locations.

DESPITE ADVANCES in our ability to diagnose and treat both acute and chronic medical conditions, we frequently fail to translate that ability into deliverable services. As a result of geographic and socio-economic constraints, thousands of Georgians, disenfranchised from the health care system, are being denied basic medical services. Providing affordable, quality health care to patients where and when they need it has remained a frustratingly elusive goal. One of the major barriers to health care for patients in isolated or impoverished communities is the inadequate number of physicians who choose to establish or maintain their practice outside of a major metropolitan area. This resulting lack of physicians in Georgia's more isolated communities compromises both quality and continuity of care. Transportation costs also increase as patients must be transferred to distant hospitals. These transfers are deleterious not only to the patient but to the community as well. As a local hospital's bed census declines, its fiscal viability, along with the socio-economic fabric of the community, is threatened.

Clearly, innovative alternatives to the existing health care delivery system must be developed, implemented, and evaluated. Georgia's isolated communities need a health care system that brings together existing professional and technologic resources to meet patients' medical needs. This alternative system needs to have the capacity to disperse and decentralize resources without compromising quality of care or escalating costs.

Committed to alleviating Georgia's health care delivery crisis, the Medical College of Georgia (MCG) developed and implemented a medical network known as the Telemedicine System. Introduced in November, 1991, and operating at MCG, the Telemedicine System effectively narrows the gap between our medical expertise and our health care delivery system. Using an interactive voice and color video telecommunication system integrated with biomedical telemetry, physicians at a medical hub, such as MCG, can examine and treat patients at multiple satellite locations, e.g., rural hospitals, ambulatory health centers, nursing homes, emergency rooms, correctional institutions, and international health facilities. By electronically transporting the expertise and state of the art technology of a major medical center to an isolated community, the Telemedicine System enhances patient care. When this System is utilized, patients can receive optimum medical care in their local hospital, avoiding both the costs and emotional distress of travel to a distant hospital. By remaining in their community, the patient also benefits from the continuity of care offered by their own physician. In cases of trauma, the Telemedicine System can decrease both morbidity and mortality by bringing immediate, state-of-the-art, trauma care to the injured patient.

By providing consultation, technologic services, and continuing medical education, the Telemedicine System also enhances the capabilities of local physicians. This, in turn, reduces their malpractice exposure and diminishes their sense of professional isolation. These benefits encourage physicians to establish and maintain practices in our smaller, rural communities. An increase in the number of physicians translates not only into better medical care for patients but also into economic growth for

Dr Sanders is Director of the Telemedicine Center Medical College of Georgia, and Dr Tedesco is President of MCG. Send reprint requests to Dr Sanders at MCG, Augusta, GA 30912-1655

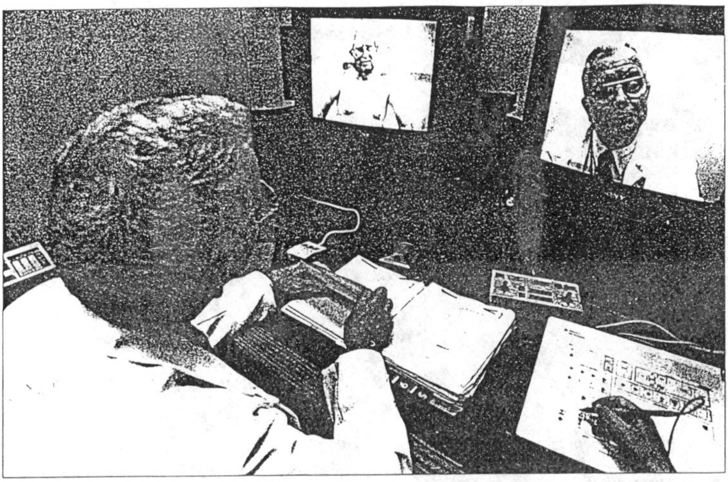

Using the Telemedicine System. Dr. Marshall B. Allen, Chief of Neurosurgery at the Medical College of Georgia, conducts a consultation with a patient at a satellite location.

hospitals and the communities they serve. When revenues generated in meeting the health care needs of local residents remain in the community, everyone benefits.

The Telemedicine System is effective with virtually any medical specialty. Based on the requirements of the satellite location, any number of diagnostic devices can be integrated into the system. The physician at the medical hub can conduct a complete history and physical examination as if the patient at the satellite location were sitting in his/her office. The remotely controlled examination camera has a powerful zoom-focus capability, enabling a dermatologist to examine minute details of a patient's skin. An electronic stethoscope, in conjunction with real-time digital transmission of an EKG or echocardiogram, enables a cardiologist to conduct a complete cardiac examination.

Specific camera adapters and resolution capabilities enhanced by remote controlled optics, provide the ophthalmologist a clear view of the retina of a patient who may be miles away. An ENT specialist can observe a laryngoscopic examination. A gastroenterologist can direct an endoscopic procedure. A radiologist can interpret x-ray findings, including MRIs, CAT scans, and ultrasound. A pathologist, utilizing the telemicroscopic adaptor, can examine a frozen section or bone marrow slide. A surgeon or gynecologist can guide a laparoscopic procedure.

In addition to directly examining and treating patients, specialists at a medical hub can also provide assistance and ongoing training to physicians at a satellite location. A thoracic surgeon can guide a local surgeon performing thoracoscopic surgery. A urologist can monitor a cystoscopic procedure; an orthopedist can direct arthroscopic surgery. A trauma surgeon at a medical hub can examine an accident victim at a satellite location and then guide the local medical team as they carry out resuscitative measures and surgical procedures.

At the heart of the Telemedicine System is a computer controlled switching matrix that allows networking between the medical hub and multiple satellite locations. If desired, the video component of the System can tape consultations for record keeping, quality assessment, and teaching purposes. A high speed, plain paper facsimile affords immediate, efficient document transfer of patient records, prescriptions, consultation notes, data base references, etc.

Freeze-frame capability allows any image projected at either the medical hub or satellite location to be "frozen" and sent as a slide to the other facility. With a special menu provided by the control panel, x-rays, EKGs, and slides can be annotated with an electronic pen. An x-ray can be viewed on one video monitor while the patient examination is viewed on a second monitor. And as the specialist at the medical hub and the treating physician at the satellite location can evaluate the patient simultaneously, the latter physician receives

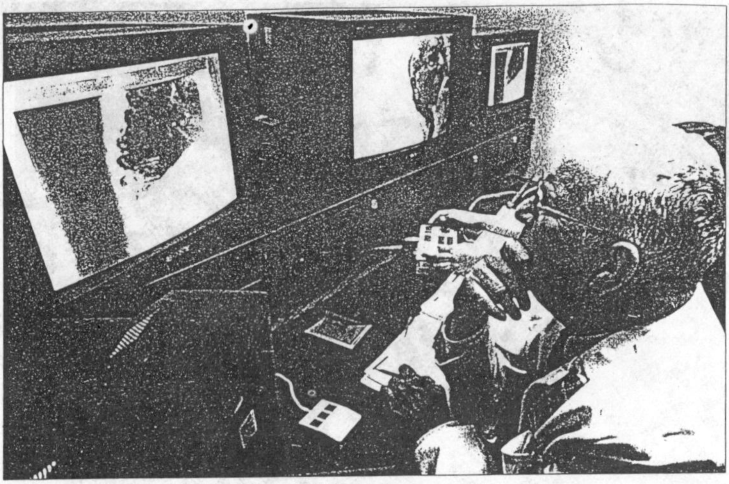

an immediate interactive educational experience that would not otherwise be available.

As a result of these interactive consultations, the expertise of local physicians is enhanced, enabling them to handle increasingly more complex problems. By sharing with physicians in isolated communities the expertise and technology available at major medical hubs, the Telemedicine System ensures that the latest advances in diagnosis and treatment are made available to all Georgians. The goal of The Telemedicine System is to assure that everyone in our state, whether living in the heart of Atlanta or on a south Georgia farm, has immediate access to quality medical care.

When patients are treated in their own community rather than transferred to a regional hospital, their physicians are able to provide continuity of care. In those instances where patient transfer is indicated, the local physician receives continual updates from the medical hub. Then when the patient is ready for discharge, the System provides the local physician with the expertise and technology needed to render follow-up treatment. For the patient, this means they are not further burdened with additional transportation costs of repeated trips back to the medical hub. In addition to saving both time and money, the patient is also able to conserve energy, typically in low reserve after a serious illness or injury.

A major benefit of the Telemedicine System is cost containment. The cost of a consult over the System is comparable to that of an EKG or chest x-ray. However, a decrease in total expenditures occurs due to the decline in patient transfers. This savings results from decreased transportation costs as well as the cost differential between the two types of facilities. Though overall costs are reduced, revenues that are generated remain within the patient's community. Keeping health care dollars in the community encourages physicians to continue practicing in the area. This, in turn, strengthens the revenue base of the community hospital, enhancing quality of care while reducing per-patient costs. And as the health care industry is frequently a major employer in rural areas, the entire community can benefit from economic growth.

The medical hub requires space comparable to the total square footage of a physician's office. Space requirements for the satellite location are equivalent to a physician's examination room. The Telemedicine System is compatible with multiple types of communication systems: telephone, cable, microwave, satellite. The full complement of equipment needed by both the medical hub and its satellite locations can be easily installed and, as the need arises, relocated.

Adaptable to a mobile configuration, the equipment can also be placed in a small van and taken to multiple sites. This flexibility enables a satellite location to have access to specialty equipment on an as needed basis. Another advantage of the Telemedicine System is its almost limitless range. Once hooked up to the System, a cardiologist in Atlanta would be able to examine the heart of a patient across the country or across the street.

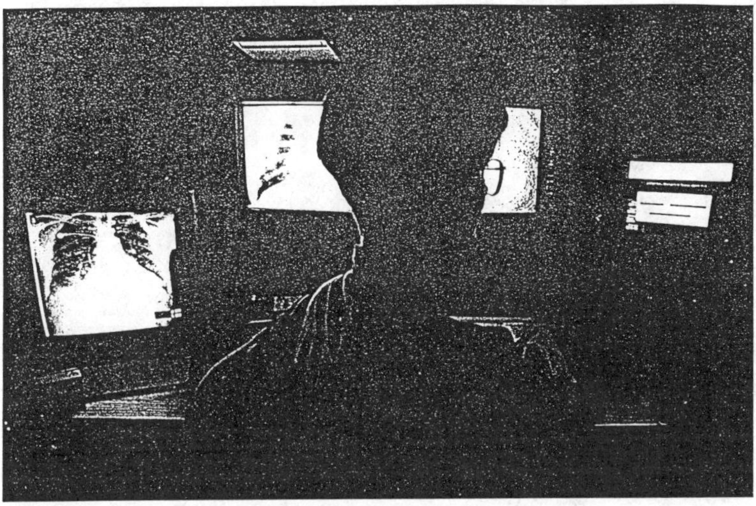

Elizabeth Michael, the Telemedicine Coordinator, studies patient test results in the Telemedicine Center

The impact of the Telemedicine System has been so significant in the Augusta region that the Medical College of Georgia is proposing to Governor Miller that it be replicated statewide. We envision the state being divided into 6-8 regions that parallel existing medical (trauma network) and communication (LATA) boundaries.

Each medical hub would be charged with the responsibility for providing consultation and technologic assistance to all under-served health care facilities in their region. This would include, in addition to isolated hospitals, public health clinics, correctional institutions, and nursing homes. We will propose to the Governor that he charge a designated state agency or a public-private partnership group with the responsibility of establishing the criteria a health care facility would need to meet in order to be included in the network.

We will ask that this designated agency or group also be charged with the responsibility of establishing and maintaining a digital telecommunication system that links each hub to their area health care facilities and to each other. Additional responsibilities that would appropriately fall to the designated agency include purchasing, integrating, and maintaining the system. This would involve assuring system component compatibility, assessing new technologies for system integration and assuring multipoint switching capability. Finally, we will ask the Governor to appoint regional quality assurance committees, composed of physicians, patients, and other community professionals, to monitor the System's quality, accessibility and affordability.

By adopting this System statewide, Georgia has a unique opportunity to enhance medical services while simultaneously lowering costs and advancing economic development in our more isolated areas. By providing immediate access to quality health care services, the System alleviates many of the problems we confront in our efforts to bring technology and expertise to the people we took an oath to care for. The Telemedicine System puts quality medical care within reach of geographically and socio-economically isolated patients. By fostering continuing education, the System also markedly diminishes the sense of professional isolation physicians in rural communities often experience. And when patients are able to remain in their local hospital, they benefit from both the medical and psychologic advantages that continuity of care by one's own physician inherently confers.

The Telemedicine System exemplifies how the introduction of new technology can expand the availability and accessibility of medical care. With increased access to medical services, Georgians can become healthier and the overall burden on our health care system can be subsequently diminished. As local medical facilities become better able to care for patients, more physicians and health care dollars will remain in these smaller, more isolated communities. The Telemedicine System has the capacity to take Georgia's health care delivery system into the 21st century; and in so doing, point the way for the nation.

Bibliography

1. Robert Wood Johnson Foundation. Access to health care in the United States: Results of a 1986 survey (special report 2). Princeton: Robert Wood Johnson Foundation 1987.

2. Butler PA. Too poor to be sick. Access to medical care for the uninsured. Washington, DC: American Public Health Association 1988.

3. Freeman HE. Blendon RJ. Aiken LH. Sudman S. Mullinix CF. Corey CR. Americans report on their access to health care. Health AFF (MIllwood) 1987;6:6-18.

4. Dwyer TF. Telepsychiatry. Psychiatric consultation by interactive television. Am J Psych 1973;1308:865-869.

5. Fisch A. Dwyer TF. Interactive Television in continuing education of foreign-trained Psychiatrists. J Med Ed 1972:47:912-914.

6. Murphy RLH. Bird KT. Telediagnosis: A new community health resource. Am J Public Health 64:113-119.

7. Sanders JH, Sasmor L. Telecommunications in health care delivery. National Science Foundation. Proceedings of the First Symposium on RANN 1973:167-169.

8. Gross CM, Ward DF, Grace R. Sanders JH. Rogers WB. Long-distance digital transmission of real-time and video taped echocardiographic images. Annual Scientific Meeting, American Society of Echocardiography. (abstract) Boston. MA. 1992

* * *

In vain do they talk of happiness who never subdued an impulse in obedience to a principle. He who never sacrificed a present to a future good, or a personal to a general one, can speak of happiness only as the blind speak of color.

— HORACE MANN

Our definition of success is unorthodox. We claim that any man who is honest, fair, tolerant, kindly, charitable of others and well behaved is a success, no matter what his station in life.

— JAY E. HOUSE

What is difficulty? Only a word indicating the degree of strength requisite for accomplishing particular objects; a mere notice of the necessity for exertion; a bugbear to children and fools; only a mere stimulus to men.

— SAMUEL WARREN

Temptation rarely comes in working hours. It is in their leisure time that men are made or marred.

— W.M. TAYLOR

Head knowledge is good, but heart knowledge is indispensable. The training of the hands and feet must be added to make a rounded education. We must all learn these days to become spiritual pioneers if we would save the world from chaos.

— E.V. HAMMOND

The functions of an executive are to create and enforce policies rather than to work out problems resulting from such policies.

— LOUIS F. MUSIL

Gaiety that sweetens existence and makes it wholesome — a sense of humor, a zest of enjoyment — this is the accompaniment of courage which gives it a supreme value. Something of the high laughter of a Cyrano de Bergerac — the world needs it.

— DR. HEBERT HICKEN

Reprinted from pages 237-241 of the May, 1993, Journal of the Medical Association of Georgia

Mr. HAYES. Thanks very much and either of the two of you wish to proceed, the order is not very important to us.

STATEMENT OF DR. ERIC TANGALOS, M.D., ASSOCIATE PROFESSOR OF MEDICINE, MAYO CLINIC, ROCHESTER, MN

Dr. TANGALOS. I think it might be better if I went next because Dr. Gomez will take us offshore completely.

Mr. HAYES. That will be fine.

Dr. TANGALOS. Mr. Chairman, Ms. Morella, thank you very much for the opportunity to provide testimony on telemedicine. I am a primary care physician and member of Mayo Foundation's Communications Committee. My remarks will be followed by a 12-minute video demonstration of telemedicine in action.

The technology making telemedicine possible is evolving at a rapid pace, such that capabilities that seemed futuristic just a few years ago are commonplace today, and the potential uses of telemedicine are tremendous. At the same time, the need to address the enormous proportion of national resources going into medical care in the U.S. and the inequities in access to care among different parts of our populations has reached a critical stage.

It is important to America that national communications policy encourage all providers to deploy services and support where it is most needed. The promise of telemedicine is to serve the underserved.

My involvement in telemedicine has already taken me beyond the high tech and highly supportive environment of the Mayo Clinic. The practice of medicine is carried out to lesser degrees in underserved and rural environments, and in inner-city hospitals and clinics that overwhelm those who choose to serve.

Globally, other countries struggle with adequate phone service to address their telemedicine needs. In the Third World, establishing a satisfactory local dial tone is far more critical than communicating with the low orbit satellite bridging two continents.

The information highway is going to have some very congested cloverleafs. It is also going to have an awful lot of dirt roads. Health system reform has access as its major priority, but it also talks about new incentives to deliver care.

The same is true for our emerging communications policy. Rural and underserved communities have just about as much success in attracting technology as they do medical services. Just as we have defined urban and rural health professional shortage areas and have provided bonuses these past five years to facilitate access to care for underserved medicare beneficiaries, carriers must also have new incentives to deploy fiber, equipment, and service to those communities that neither command market share or capital to stand on their own.

It is unfortunate because of our internal barriers and policy limitations, telemedicine may be easier to carry out beyond our own national boundaries. Just recently rural health initiatives in Alaska have looked to Norway for solutions to their problems. Although international trade should be encouraged, it is the export of our services that should be promoted. And if we continue to tie health care costs to the Gross National Product, what better way to provide access to care at home than to fund it with the export of our expertise?

How quickly telemedicine is deployed will be determined by Congress in its support of research, demonstration projects, and a national policy which either promotes collaboration or drives private competition. Mayo may be able to establish its own network to deliver services to select sites at home and abroad, and will go head to head with for-profit subsidiaries such as Massachusetts General Hospital's American Telemedicine International in the Middle East. Projects in Oregon, Georgia, Kansas, and Iowa, have as their major goal in-State services. And exclusivity already exists in some situations to allow access to communications networks only to State-run programs in education and government.

These limitations work against physician groups not recognized as providing State-sponsored medical education or public health, telephone and cable companies, and physician practices that may see patients crossing State lines.

It should also be by congressional mandate that telemedicine projects provide a point of service option for all patients and health plans. By encouraging open systems that compete on quality and cost and are not defined by hard geographic boundaries, we can create a much more robust network with greater accessibility and the freedom of choice.

New technology that can be produced and deployed cheaply and effectively to meet economic performance standards will deliver the promise of telemedicine to health system's reform.

Acceptable standards for telemedicine activities may include the provision that less information will be available to provide care than face-to-face consultation. Effectiveness research will evaluate patient satisfaction and functional status. Utility measurements will need to focus on outcome rather than process. Clinical trials will need to be considered on their own merit, but also in the larger context of telemedicine's value to the community.

It is essential that active telemedicine programs begin to collect data in a standardized fashion so that large volumes of information can be gathered in a systematic way to guide best practice models. Programs like those at the University of Kansas have begun to look at changes in practice patterns and outcomes of care.

Although these projects have very small numbers, this type of activity will provide the credibility to substantiate telemedicine as a new paradigm to deliver medical care.

The institution of guidelines for the application of telemedicine is being quickly realized. As telemedicine appears to be on the verge of making the transition from an experimental and research technology to an applied science, there may be tremendous practical application.

The medical community, through its professional societies, as well as governmental agencies such as the Agency for Health Care Policy and Research Office of the Forum and the Health Care Financing Administration's Health Standards and Quality Bureau will be interested in such best practice models.

However, a number of universal problems will be confronted when approaching telemedicine across State lines. The first two issues are matters on which Congress might wish to consider developing some standardization. They are: One, defining situations in which licensing is required. Two, assuring compliance with licensing requirements when applicable.

The last four items are matters which more appropriately should evolve through the practice of telemedicine and do not require congressional intervention or legislative intervention. Three, determining an acceptable interface for patients from separate groups or private practices that have purchased dissimilar equipment; four, establishing criteria to engage physicians in the consultative practice of telemedicine both within an institution and in the community. Five, insuring appropriate billing mechanisms and third-party reimbursement for telemedicine consultations; and six, defining the practice parameters between providing consultative services and actual participation in a patient's care.

Government intervention at too early a stage may serve to stifle rather than foster growth and the concepts and technology needed for telemedicine to work. Both technical and practice standards for telemedicine should be established by professional medical societies. The AMA has already begun its own investigation into this emerging field and will include in its understanding of telemedicine the issues of quality and standards for care.

The American Telemedicine Association of which Jay and I are both board members is also addressing these issues.

Practitioners and patients in isolation may ultimately determine the usefulness and implementation of telemedicine. Technology vendors, health plan administrators, State health boards, and subspecialty physicians in regional medical centers are not the end users.

Given the expense involved to establish new networks of care, the measure of success may be based on community standards rather than on usual and customary medical practice. The family practitioner or public health nurse in the underserved area are the people who need to learn more about telemedicine and guide its development.

A major barrier to the utilization of telemedicine is the current failure to reach the end user with information about its potential application.

The partnerships to make telemedicine work include the patient, the health team, local, regional and long-distance carriers, and a supportive political and regulatory community. The weakest link in this partnership currently is patient understanding and consumer advocacy.

The focus for telemedicine should be on access, but the means to deliver care have not yet been clearly elucidated. Educational efforts must be undertaken to lay out the realities of the present day marketplace and the potential that exists for more fully integrated programs to bring better health to each citizen.

I would now like to share with you some telemedicine examples at my institution. You may want to move to some better seats. This will take 12 minutes and I will leave a copy of this video with Monica.

[A video was shown.]

[The prepared statement of Eric Tangalos, M.D. follows:]

Mayo Clinic/Mayo Foundation
200 First Street, SW
Rochester, MN 55905
(507) 284-5126 FAX (507) 284-5073

Hearing on TELEMEDICINE: AN INFORMATION HIGHWAY TO SAVE LIVES

SUBCOMMITTEE ON INVESTIGATIONS AND OVERSIGHT
COMMITTEE ON SCIENCE, SPACE, AND TECHNOLOGY
UNITED STATES HOUSE OF REPRESENTATIVES

MAY 2, 1994

Eric G. Tangalos, M.D.
Associate Professor of Medicine

EXECUTIVE SUMMARY

Deployment of Telemedicine

It is important to America that national communications policy encourages technology providers to deploy service and support where it is most needed. The promise of telemedicine is to serve the underserved. It must be clearly understood that there will be additive costs to delivering care to those who presently receive none or very little. This includes service to our inner cities, the home bound and the isolated. The family practitioner or public health nurse in the underserved area are the people who need to learn more about telemedicine and begin to guide its development. Telemedicine applications must be consumer driven. The practice of medicine quickly adjusts to new technology and has already embraced all of the hardware and software that goes with electronic data interchange. However, our public which is usually excited about any breakthrough product, has yet to understand the process whereby telemedicine can provide access and deliver care.

Impediments to Care

The information explosion has surpassed the capabilities of our current regulated communications network. Limitations on the business opportunities of the telephone companies -- whether bans of long distance service, research, design and manufacturing, or interactive video services -- result in patients and healthcare professionals not having the full range of products and services that should be available to them. One of the most difficult hurdles to surmount is connectivity, between local and long distance carriers. The current interLATA restrictions greatly reduce flexibility, responsiveness and creativity. A major barrier to the utilization of telemedicine is the current failure to reach the end user with information about its potential applications.

Policy Issues for Congress

How quickly telemedicine is deployed will be determined by Congress in its support of research, demonstration projects and a national policy which either promotes collaboration or drives private competition. It should also be by congressional mandate that telemedicine projects provide a point of service option for all patients and health plans. By encouraging open systems that compete on quality and cost and are not defined by hard geographic boundaries, we can create a much more robust network with greater accessibility and the freedom of choice. The partnerships to make telemedicine work include the patient, the health care team, local regional and long-distance carriers, and a supportive political and regulatory community. The focus may be on access, but the means to deliver care have not been clearly elucidated. New technology that can be produced and deployed cheaply and effectively to meet economic performance standards will deliver the promise of telemedicine to health care reform.

Reimbursement

An underlying issue that must be addressed before telemedicine can be fully utilized is reimbursement for the medical care which involves advanced communication networks. Currently, only technology-based information transfer (e.g. - reading of transmitted radiological images) is routinely reimbursed by federally-funded health care programs such as Medicare. Many questions must be addressed before this coverage will be offered by regional carriers and third party payers. For example, can the usual requirement for "face-to-face" contact between physician and patient be modified? Is the quality of care provided via telemedicine up to standards of the medical community? The Health Care Financing Administration rightfully asks for outcome studies as it plans its strategy to pay for services but may hold telemedicine to greater scrutiny than what currently defines the daily practice of medicine. There is great hesitancy on the part of many providers to enter the practice of telemedicine given the uncertainty of how these services are to be recognized and reimbursed.

Medicine's Initiatives

The history of telemedicine is relatively short, dating back only to about 1959. As with many new technologies, it has struggled with changing (improving) technology, costs associated with new ideas, and acceptance of new approaches by people accustomed to set ways. As one reviews the literature, however, it is striking how the vast majority of patients and practitioners who actually experience telemedicine find it to be effective and useful. The major focus of these experiments has been on telemedicine as a vehicle for extending high quality medical care to people in remote areas to improve available care and minimize the travel time of health care providers. Rural states have taken the lead in establishing programs to serve the rural and underserved and are supported by federal agencies such as the REA. The Agency for Health Care Policy and Research helped fund a consensus conference carried out during the first *Mayo Telemedicine Symposium*. The consensus statement outlining the guiding principles for the use of telecommunications technologies in the delivery of medical care and information can be found in the body of this report.

WRITTEN TESTIMONY

Policy

The technology making telemedicine possible is evolving at a very rapid pace, such that capabilities that seemed futuristic a few years ago are commonplace today, and the potential uses of telemedicine are tremendous. At the same time, the need to address the enormous proportion of national resources going into medical care in the U.S., and the inequities in the access to care among different parts of our population, has reached a critical stage.

My involvement in telemedicine has already taken me beyond the high tech and highly supportive environment of Mayo Clinic. The practice of medicine is carried out to lesser degrees in underserved and rural environments and in inner city hospitals and clinics that overwhelm those who choose to serve. Globally, other countries struggle with adequate phone service to address their telemedicine needs. In the third world establishing a satisfactory local dial tone is far more critical than communicating with the low orbit satellite bridging two continents.

Washington's responsibility to sovereign nations need not go beyond our own shores. The Bureau of Indian Affairs and the Indian Health Service struggle with some of the most difficult health care needs and inaccessible populations we ever face. Our history of help with these populations remains poor. Demonstration projects and worthwhile experiments crisscross the landscape of the Indian nation, yet sustainable programs both in health care and industry are few and far between. The American markets are not at Pine Ridge or Red Lake. We choose, instead, to compete for medical and communication services in our major metropolitan areas.

The information highway is going to have some very congested cloverleafs. Its also going to have an awful lot of dirt road. Health system reform has access as its major priority, but it also talks about new incentives to deliver care. The same is true for our emerging communication policy. Carriers must have new incentives to deploy fiber, equipment and service to those communities that neither command market share or capital to stand on their own. Rural and underserved communities have just about as much success in attracting technology as they do medical service. Other countries choose to reward cooperation more than competition and in so doing link health care, education and community development in more affordable and satisfying ways.

Telemedicine in Norway is probably the most developed in the world. The first tests were carried out by the Norwegian Telecom Research, and in 1986, an initiative was taken in Finmark with a project called "Telematics in Finmark's Public Health Service". The political reality was that new technical developments could contribute to the security and improve the public health service. This realization was endorsed by the government through the resolutions "National Plan of Action for Information Technology in 1986 and Growth and New Development in the North 1987". In 1991, the project "Telemedicine in Nordland" was started as a direct consequence of a political decision: that all hospitals in the country shall remain operative. The Norwegian program combines the elements of medicine and communications and has a complete network of initiatives and activities. In particular, the University Hospital of Tromso has served as a focal point for these activities.[1]

It is important to America that national communications policy encourages technology providers to deploy service and support where it is most needed. The information explosion has surpassed the capabilities of our current regulated communications network. Limitations on the business opportunities of the telephone companies -- whether bans of long distance service, research, design and manufacturing, or interactive video services -- result in patients and healthcare professionals not having the full range of products and services that should be available to them. One of the most difficult hurdles to surmount is connectivity, between local and long distance carriers. The current interLATA restrictions greatly reduce flexibility, responsiveness and creativity.

Similarly, other government restrictions and regulatory rules impede the deployment of new technologies and provide very little incentive for telephone companies to invest in new networks that would improve the opportunities to fully utilize telemedicine. The piece work that now goes on to make systems work is costly, ineffecient and hightly technical. A recent Wall Street Journal article (April 8, 1994) noted that the FCC "has just apporved five trials for interactive video services. Another 17 requests are pending, and some of them have languished at the agency for more than a year." My telemedicine colleagues are not waiting on ATM, fiber or satellite hubs for their campuses, what they want now are better rates and a level of service that would make their telemedicine projects part of a routine and not exceptions to the rule.

A major barrier to the utilization of telemedicine is the current failure to reach the end user with information about its potential applications. Technology vendors, healthplan administrators, state health administrators, and subspecialty physicians in regional medical centers are not the end users. The family practitioner or public health nurse in the underserved area are the people who need to learn more about telemedicine and begin to guide its development.

It is unfortunate that because of our internal barriers and policy limitations telemedicine may be easier to carry out beyond our national boundaries. Just recently rural health initiatives in Alaska have looked to Norway for solutions to their problems. Although international trade should be encouraged, it is the export of our services that should be promoted. And if we continue to tie health care costs to the Gross National Product what better way to provide access to care at home than to fund it with the export of our expertise. The promise of telemedicine is to serve the underserved, there will be additive costs to delivering care to those who presently receive no care or very little care in our inner cities or are home bound and isolated.

How quickly telemedicine is deployed will be determined by Congress in its support of research, demonstration projects and a national policy which either promotes collaboration or drives private competition. Mayo may be able to establish its own network to deliver services to select sites at home and abroad and will go head to head with for profit subsidiaries such as Massachusetts General Hospital's American Telemedicine International in the Middle East. Projects in Oregon, Georgia, Kansas and Iowa have as their major goal in-state services. This exclusivity goes as far as to consider only state run programs in education and government, often to the disadvantage to our Regional Bell Operating Companies and independent TELCOs. Also disadvantaged are physician groups not recognized as state sponsored education programs or government health care providers. In the vernacular of health system reform it will by congressional mandate to provide a point of service option for our patients and health plans. By encouraging open systems that compete on quality and cost which are not defined by hard geographic boundaries, we can create a much more robust network with greater accessibility and the freedom of choice.

Applications

Telecommunications in medicine takes a number of different forms, but in each case requires a method for producing an audiovisual signal at one site, converting that signal to a transmissible signal, transmission, receiving the signal, and reconverting it to a usable format. In some cases, such as in some education programs, it is not necessary for the receiving site to be able to transmit both audio and video response; questions can be posed to a presenter via telephone. In many cases, especially with medical treatments, true two-way audiovisual linkage is essential. Signals are transmitted via analog or digital format using either satellite or, more recently, fiber optic cable. One of the limiting factors to dissemination of telemedicine, until recently, has been the size and cost of the technology. Dramatic improvements in the past few years, along with improved transmission capabilities via satellite, fiber optics and copper wire, have brought the technology much closer to practicality for many small medical centers and rural locations. In these days of compressed video at quarter T1 and below, projections of the continued improvements in technology clearly show that cost-effectiveness is close at hand.

The history of telemedicine is relatively short, dating back only to about 1959[2] and could be described as a series of exploratory pilot projects with limited long-term continuity. As with many new technologies, it has struggled with changing (improving) technology, costs associated with new ideas, and acceptance of new approaches by people accustomed to set ways. As one reviews the literature, however, it is striking how the vast majority of patients and practitioners who actually experience telemedicine find it to be effective and useful. The major focus of these experiments has been on telemedicine as a vehicle for extending high quality medical care to people in remote areas to improve available care and minimize the travel time of health care providers. Clearly, it has the potential to play an important role in such situations.

The longest-running effective use of telemedicine appears to be in Australia and Canada, likely locations due to the large, sparsely populated land areas separating population centers Early demonstration projects in Australia[3] showed how effective satellite-based telemedicine could be. Similarly, Canadian groups effectively use telemedicine to provide both medical care and continuing medical education to remote sites.[4,5,6,7] Several projects in the U.S. also have shown some effective use of telemedicine. Most recently, two separate projects in Texas (Texas Tech Med Net, recently renamed Health Net, and the Texas Telemedicine Project) are evaluating the effective use of telemedicine to improve care in small cities at modest distances from major medical centers. Projects from Montana, Kansas, Georgia, North Carolina, and other states are currently looking at applications of telemedicine as well.

Telemedicine applications must be consumer driven. The practice of medicine quickly adjusts to new technology and has already embraced all of the hardware and software that goes with electronic data interchange. However, our public which is usually excited about any breakthrough product, has yet to understand the process whereby telemedicine can provide access to care and deliver it as well. The "electronic house call" and "telehealth" have yet to enter the daily dictionary of health system reform. Will the public believe that this technology will improve quality while at the same time reducing cost? Will projects under development avoid hospitalizations for at risk groups through active intervention? What level of investment will institutions make in planning their own futures? At Mayo all three group practice sites are actively pursuing the implementation of an Electronic Medical Record (EMR).

A planning task force for a Mayo EMR completed its work in December 1992 and an implementation work group in Rochester has been active for eighteen months. Jacksonville has begun a pilot of an EMR in workstation concepts which will include portable devices and voice recognition. The Jacksonville clinic is also relying more on outside vendors for support than is occurring with the development taking place on the Rochester campus. Communication of EMR related data with affiliated rural practices is also under development. It is our belief that the medical environment of the future will be electronic thus permitting greater efficiencies and accuracy.

Research

One very important issue in comparing technologies is the quality of audio and video signals. In full-motion telemedicine the quality of sound and picture are equivalent to the highest qualities currently seen in television transmissions. To minimize costs of transmission, "compressed" signals can be transmitted at lower costs but with varying degrees of fidelity. The biggest loss of fidelity comes as subjects move, generating a jerky appearance and substantial time delays. For static events or low rates of movement these signals can still be quite satisfactory. Mayo's research interests in telemedicine allow us to more quickly evaluate developing technologies and the strategies necessary for institutions to integrate services along new information highways.

It is essential that active telemedicine programs begin to collect data in a standardized fashion so that larger volumes of information can be gathered in a systematic way to guide best practice models. Programs like those at the University of Kansas[8] have begun to look at changes in practice patterns and outcomes of care. Although these projects have very small numbers this type of activity will provide the credibility to substantiate telemedicine as a new paradigm to deliver medical care.

Unfortunately, the literature is devoid of outcome studies or health care effectiveness research. Given the lengthy adolescence of telemedicine, most published accounts on direct physician to patient interactions are descriptive or at best evaluative. None of the projects have gone into great detail to use the framework of Structure, Process and Outcome. In today's vernacular of health care reform the terms would be Access, Quality and Cost, but the rigors for scientific investigation should be the same. Specific aims need to be established for investigators to use appropriate materials and methods to measure and evaluate results. Conflicts are sure to arise if policy and practice rush ahead of cost effectiveness and practical economics.

Standards to measure technical image quality have only been described in radiology, yet here the process is well underway.[9] Radiologist performance has been tested comparing plain film interpretation against digitized images on a video monitor[10] and laser-digitized workstation images sent on T1 lines have been compared against conventional analog radiographs.[11] In the latter study 40 pneumonia and 40 trauma cases were compared to controls to develop a receiver operating characteristic (ROC) analysis.

In 1982, the American College of Radiology (ACR) and the National Electrical Manufacturers Association (NEMA) formed a Committee to develop standards for communications between medical imaging devices. Versions 1.0 and 2.0 published in 1985 and 1988 respectively, were concerned with point-to-point image transmission, while Version 3.0, also referred to as DICOM, provides specifications for network connections. The DICOM Standard conforms to the International Standards Organizations (ISO) reference model for network communications, maintains compatibility with the earlier point-to-point Versions 1. and 2., and incorporates the concept of object-oriented design.[12]

Both for transmission and storage purposes, information preserving data compression algorithms are required which are optimized for medical imagery (not for consumer viewing, as is now the case). In an article published in the SMPTE Journal[13], Mayo

Foundation described the technical findings of a study whose purpose was to determine the utility of compressed video techniques for video conferencing and medical diagnostic image consultation. Mayo Foundation has experimented with several commercially available image compression algorithms, and has found that critical fine detail is not preserved by these algorithms. A wide bandwidth satellite video conferencing system has been implemented at Ku band and utilized for teleconferencing and medical diagnostic consultation since 1986 between the three facilities which comprise the Mayo Foundation. This study was conducted to determine which, if any, of the currently available video compression techniques could serve as an alternative to the wideband satellite communications modality.

Radiology's need to communicate has been moved along by interest in the picture archiving and communication systems (PACS) and are under development at many major medical centers. The design for global communications networks is well underway and the remote consultation and diagnosis operation has been tested in real time between the University Medical Center in Tucson, Arizona, and the Bowman Gray School of Medicine at Wake Forest University using Internet. In the remote consultation and diagnosis operation, a set of images is requested from the database archives system and the image is sent to the local and remote work station sites on a Global PACS network. Future improvements to the system will include real-time voice and interactive compressed video scenarios in the use of ATM/SONET communications systems.[14]

There is already an ongoing debate regarding data transmission with compression where there is no loss of image and where there is some loss of image. Telepathology is generally limited to local area network and relies principally on analog video signals. Some of the earliest work dates back to 1987.[15] The University of Arizona at Tucson has considered the quality of the video image with regard to three factors: 1) image fidelity; 2) informativeness; and 3) aesthetics. A purely physical method such as measuring the signal-to-noise characteristics of a video monitor can be used to assess image fidelity; but well controlled observer performance studies must be conducted to assess the ways in which image informativeness and aesthetics influence diagnostic accuracy.[16] Whereas dynamic (real-time) telepathology imaging requires the use of broad-band telecommunications channels, static telepathology imaging can be carried out over conventional telephone lines. Several studies have measured viewing times per case and diagnostic accuracy. Results indicate that viewing times are increased fivefold or more with static imaging compared with real time dynamic imaging.[17] Weinstein et. al. suggest that combining slow-scan real time imaging, for specimen orientation, with static imaging may not improve viewing times over those obtained with static imaging alone. It goes on to point out the diagnostic accuracy may be similar with static and dynamic imaging.

Currently most pathology applications of telemedicine are used as back up and confirmation of an on-site primary diagnosis. As the applications for telepathology increase and more responsibility is required of a singular pathologist to stand by a diagnosis, standards will be invoked to protect against malpractice. Services such as emergency care, surgery, dermatology, cardiology, psychiatry and medical consultation will require further scrutiny. Although investigations began as long as 20 years ago studying the effectiveness of cardiac auscultation via microwave transmission[18] recent outcomes work has not been published. In most cases the delivery of telemedicine services serve as a back up to practitioners on the front lines.

Standards of Care

Acceptable standards for telemedicine activities may include the provision that less information will be available to provide care than face-to-face in-person consultation. Effectiveness research will evaluate patient satisfaction and functional status. Utility measurements will need to focus on outcome rather than process. Clinical trials will need to be considered on their own merit but also in the larger context of telemedicine's value to the community.

The institution of guidelines for the application of telemedicine is being quickly realized. As telemedicine appears to be on the verge of making the transition from an experimental and research technology to an applied science, there may be tremendous practical application. The medical community through its professional societies as well as governmental agencies such as the Agency for Health Care Policy and Research Office of the Forum and the Health Care Financing Administration's Health Standards and Quality Bureau will be interested in best practice models.

However, a number of universal problems will be confronted when approaching telemedicine across state lines. The first two issues are matters on which Congress might wish to consider developing some standardization. The last four items are matters which more appropriately should evolve through the practice. They are:

1. Defining situations in which licensing is required;

2. Assuring compliance with licensing requirements when applicable;

3. Determining an acceptable interface for patients from separate groups or private practices that have purchased dissimilar equipment.

4. Establishing criteria to engage physicians in the consultative practice of telemedicine both within an institution and in the community;

5. Insuring appropriate billing mechanisms and third-party reimbursement for telemedicine consultations;

6. Defining the practice parameters between providing consultative services and actual participation in a patient's care.

Government intervention at too early a stage may server to stifle rather than foster growth of the concepts and technology needed for telemedicine to work. Both technical and practice standards for telemedicine should be established by professional medical societies. The AMA has already begun its own investigation into this emerging field and will include in its understanding of telemedicine the issues of quality of care and standards for care. The American Telemedicine Association of which I am a board member is also approaching the broad question of standards.

The specific question of liability should depend on the degree to which the telemedicine consultant assumes the diagnosis and treatment of the patient. For example, for primary interpretation of teleradiology, the telemedicine radiologist is legally responsible. For consultative interpretation the responsibility is shared. The Norwegian comparison can again be stressed: There is only one payer for health in Norway and only one telecommunications company. The concept of liability is poorly developed while the concept of responsibility pervades the land and the practice of medicine.

There is a legacy of licensing and reimbursement barriers which are impediments to telemedicine. These include closed panel HMO capitation, UPIN #, and individual hospital credentials. It is not practical for consulting physicians to obtain multiple state medical licenses in order to do telemedicine regionally or nationally. As an alternative to the usual state licensing process, a national medical license limited to telemedicine consultation within an area of specialty expertise has been suggested.

We will eventually establish boundaries for an episode of care that will include telemedicine as part of the technology available to practitioners. Standards will define the process, provide uniformity, set benchmarks and develop scenarios. In the current context of recognizing services this will likely result in CPT code modifiers. One must also caution that we may be asking more of telemedicine to demonstrate effectiveness and efficacy than anything so far brought to the practice of medicine. Outcome studies are still quite limited and medical economists relatively scarce. Practice guidelines are currently in vogue but telemedicine has no history or literature of any size for comparison. It can not be evaluated as a new medical technology or procedure as it brings together basic communication technologies now better refined. It is the high visibility and obtrusive nature of the video camera and historical documentation by video tape that takes these interchanges to heights vastly different from the telephone call or informal "curbside consultation" done at medical centers and hospitals in urban settings.

Reimbursement

An underlying issue that must be addressed before telemedicine can be fully utilized is reimbursement for the medical care which involves advanced communication networks. Currently, only technology-based information transfer (e.g. - reading of transmitted radiological images) is routinely reimbursed by federally-funded health care programs such as Medicare. The Medical College of Georgia's demonstration and approved Medicare coverage by Aetna and Medicaid coverage by the state is the notable clinical exception.

Many questions must be addressed before this coverage will be offered by other regional carriers. For example, can the usual requirement for "face-to-face" contact between physician and patient be modified? Is the quality of care provided via telemedicine up to standards of the medical community? Do research findings from studies in one discipline provide information on suitability in other specialties?

As specialized care is forced to retreat in the drive toward more preventive and primary care it will become more concentrated in urban areas. The opportunities for telemedicine to provide access to consulting physicians for evaluation and management services at great distances is exciting. To maintain the highest skills for a referral practice physicians prefer a concentration of patients with a defined set of problems for which they can serve as expert help. Using secondary and tertiary care in this manner should be an efficient and cost effective way to allow specialists to practice just within their field of interest.

The cost of telemedicine should be linked to the alternative cost of transportation of moving the patient to the regional referral center for consultation. Health plans will need to consider the transportation costs for each patient referred for a face-to-face consultation versus the cost of a telemedicine consultation. By linking these two costs, health plans will be motivated to find alternative methods to deliver care to underserved areas without requiring the patient to travel. Including other telecommunications applications such as in business, education and library, will reduce the initial capital cost of establishing the telecommunication network infrastructure for telemedicine.

Implementation

A major barrier to the utilization of telemedicine is the current failure to reach the end user with information about its potential applications. Technology vendors, health plan administrators, state health administrators, and subspecialty physicians in regional medical centers are not the end users. The family practitioner or public health nurse in the underserved area are the people to who need to learn more about telemedicine and begin to guide its development.

The implications telemedicine has to the health care reform debate are significant. In general, the conceptual framework we use in this debate is a fee for service environment. If the Administration's Health Security Act of 1993 is successful at providing basic coverage and access to all Americans, then telemedicine can be a part of the solution. The paradigm will also take us more closely to a managed care environment where the solutions to problems of access and delivery reside with accountable plans more likely to embrace new technologies for the delivery of services.

Practitioners and patients in isolation may ultimately determine the usefulness and implementation of telemedicine. Given the expense involved to establish new networks of care, the measure of success may be based on community standards rather than usual and customary medical practice. Capital outlays may force mixed services including educational and administrative functions to run in parallel with patient care. Health care reform may allow calculations for travel and lost time to be included in a more global understanding of budget and costs.

Telemedicine at Mayo

Telemedicine at Mayo Clinic has evolved for very unique reasons. Mayo was involved in early experimentation with telemedicine, but became a major developer when it decided to expand out of Rochester, Minnesota, and open group practices in Scottsdale, Arizona and Jacksonville, Florida. It was established from the beginning that the group practice sites would be parts of a fully integrated system which maintained all of the strengths of the initial single site. By the time the two new group practices began operating in 1987 a fully-functional two-way telecommunications system was up and running. In 1987 the only feasible transmission modality was satellite and the only acceptable signal full motion analog video. Today, telemedicine for clinical care, education, and administrative coordination is a common, everyday, event at Mayo. The institution has purchased three transponders on the aging telecommunications satellite G-Star III to carry out two simultaneous broadcasts at all three group practice sites. The system at Mayo is a high-end, full function system which provides communication almost indistinguishable from in-person interactions.

To date Mayo has gained experience in the consultative practice of telemedicine with services limited to the three group practice sites. However, projects and grants are planned or underway to explore the direct delivery of services to our regional practice sites and beyond. These projects include the use of satellite communications to deliver consultative care to the Middle East and the use of compressed video and land lines to deliver a wide range of services to affiliated entities within the states of Iowa and Wisconsin as well as Minnesota. A contract with Amman Diagnostic Clinic in Jordan was signed in February 1994 and Mayo has participated with US West on the COMPASS trials as well as with the REA and the Office of Rural Health Policy for telemedicine workshops in 1993.

The Advanced Communications and Technology Satellite (ACTS) launched in July of 1993 has Mayo as an active investigator for much of the two years currently funded for the project. Experiments will include both T1 and high data rate terminals made available through NASA and the Advanced Research Project Agency. Because fiber land lines may not reach small communities for many years, satcom technology, such as that represented by ACTS, is a possible alternate implementation. For this reason, Mayo Foundation is already planning and executing telemedicine experiments using both the LDR and HDR features of ACTS. Mayo may also gain access to the MAGIC test bed in an attempt to mix transmission modalities for the delivery of services from a tertiary care center to far more remote environments.

Mayo Telemedicine Symposium

The first Mayo Telemedicine Symposium was held October 1-3, 1993. I was privileged to serve as course director for this program. The planning of this event began 18 months earlier and at a time before the information highway had experienced any traffic. Moreover, compression technologies now so common to the field were still very developmental and for the most part not acceptable for patient care activities. Be it foresight, timing or extremely good luck the program came off at just the right time.

The over 400 registrants who attended the symposium at the three Mayo group practice sites of Rochester, Minnesota, Jacksonville, Florida, and Scottsdale, Arizona, were included in all of the three-way programming and plenary sessions of the Symposium via the Mayo full-motion satellite communications network. Speakers made presentations from all three locations in specially equipped lecture halls. The audience had its choice of geographic locations.

The Symposium provided an appropriate backdrop for the Consensus Conference "Telemedicine and Access to Care". This consensus conference was partially sponsored by the Agency for Health Care Policy and Research Small Grants Program to create a lasting record of the meeting. Through the Consensus Conference, all Symposium participants were invited to contribute to establishment of guiding principles and priorities for greater use of telemedicine to promote access to high-quality medical care for all Americans.

The Consensus Statement which follows represents the collective knowledge, perspectives and vision of the Mayo Telemedicine Symposium participants. The degree to which consensus emerged was striking; although individuals expressed differing views on the relative importance of various topics, virtually all agreed to their inclusion. What emerged from this activity is a list of principles, questions and barriers which the participants believe must be addressed. There was unanimous agreement that telemedicine can play an important cost-effective role in delivery of medical information and care to the large population of underserved Americans. A copy of the entire *Proceedings of the Mayo Telemedicine Symposium* can be obtained free from:

Richard McGee, Ph.D.
Consensus Conference Director
Department of Education Services
Mayo Clinic and Mayo Foundation
200 First St. SW
Rochester, MN 55905

Consensus Statement
Guiding Principles for the use of telecommunications technologies in the delivery of medical care and information:

1. Emphasis should be placed on the needs of underserved populations, both rural and urban

If telemedicine is to play an important role in delivery of medical care the primary goal should be to evaluate and develop the technology from the perspective of the underserved people in the U.S. Although telemedicine has many potential uses in sophisticated information transfer between major medical centers and remote regions such as space, the most important contributions will be in the improvement of services to underserved populations in rural and urban areas.

2. Analysis and development of applications should start from the consumer, both the potential patients and the healthcare care providers who serve them

Development of telemedicine applications requires effective partnerships between consumers, local and distant healthcare care providers, technology providers and companies which manage communications networks. It is important that the starting point, however, be the consumer; "what is needed and will be used" are more important questions than "what is technologically possible". Software development also must contain a strong contribution from the end-user community.

3. Telemedicine applications must be customized by community and include as many possible uses of technologies as possible

Underserved communities invariably have limited economic resources. Thus, it is critical that new technologies introduced be utilized as fully as possible. Systems which have been successful to date have effectively brought in both medical and non-medical uses of the new telecommunications capabilities.

4. Adequate training is essential during implementation of telemedicine

With the wide dissemination of computers and video systems, most people (especially young people) are comfortable with the use of telecommunications technologies. Training in the specific use of new systems is critical, however, if practitioners are to use them.

5. Communications technology and availability can be very poor and a limiting factor in rural, and even urban, underserved areas

There are still areas in the U.S. where even telephone service is not routinely available either due to low economic resources or actual absence of lines, etc. If advanced telecommunications technology is to assist these regions equal attention must be given to basic resources.

6. A decrease in a sense of isolation is a readily observable benefit of telemedicine extended to rural communities

Professional and social isolation are known to be significant contributors to dissatisfaction among healthcare providers in underserved areas. As should be expected, effective use of telemedicine has been shown to decrease feelings of isolation. The capacity to increase the willingness of providers to work in underserved areas should be a major benefit of successful telemedicine.

7. The use of telecommunications to provide preventive health education to underserved populations may be as important as the actual improvement of care provided via telemedicine

Especially in underserved areas, accurate, appropriate health education information often is difficult to obtain. A strong consensus was established that this is a very important area to explore when developing new telemedicine and elecommunications strategies. The savings in healthcare care costs via improved preventive measures is expected to be substantial.

8. When determining cost-effectiveness of new telemedicine systems and strategies it is critical to consider VALUE to the individual and the community, with costs being only one element of the equation

The value of telemedicine systems to individuals and communities can go well beyond the simple calculations of dollars saved and additional care provided. This value includes the creation of markets, which then attracts investment and delivery of goods and services to these new markets. The reality is that telecommunications technology and infrastructure is attracted to identifiable markets. Establishment of telemedicine creates the initial value observed as a new market opportunity. Coordination of telemedicine services with other community needs and resources dramatically increases the value of these systems.

9. Professional groups within the medical community should develop minimum technology standards for delivery of telemedicine

Technological standards in delivery of telemedicine are needed. Professional groups within the medical community are most capable of developing these standards. These standards, rather than focusing on the maximum capabilities available, should focus on the minimum acceptable to insure quality but minimize costs.

10. All forms of telecommunications, not just high-end video systems, should be utilized in new telemedicine applications

It is often easier to ask "what is the state of the art" than "what is the simplest system that will do the job". New video technologies using fiber optics or satellite communications can be very compelling and have tremendous capabilities. In many instances, however, simpler, less costly alternatives are available that work well for specific applications. If only the most sophisticated current technologies are explored for telemedicine it is likely that the high costs will be unacceptable. Technologies such as the telephone, computer networks, microwave, or broadcast television all should play important roles in telemedicine. The medical community, technology providers and communications companies must share the responsibility for identification of the most appropriate and cost-effective technology for each application.

11. Effective telemedicine will dramatically improve the ability of mid-level providers (e.g. physicians assistants, nurse practitioners, etc.) to participate in healthcare delivery to underserved populations

Mid-level practitioners represent an important resource for improving access to care with a lower increase in healthcare costs. Effective telemedicine will both improve the resources available to these practitioners and decrease their sense of isolation in underserved areas. Developments in telemedicine should recognize this important link and fully develop its potential.

12. Telemedicine offers both direct access to traditional Continuing Medical Education (CME) and "instantaneous" CME with every interaction between local and distant healthcare providers

Most traditional CME has focused on providers traveling to regional and national centers for their continuing education. Telemedicine affords the opportunity for one-way or interactive CME without the provider leaving the practice sites. Additionally, each interactive session between local provider and the distant consultant provides immediate, problem-based continuing education. Learning in this problem-based setting generally tends to be highly effective and efficient, and will contribute to increased quality of care.

13. As computer networks and other communications technologies develop it will be critical that they be integrated both vertically and horizontally with each other

Current hardware and software development strategies often build upon competition rather than cooperation between developers. Although recognizing the value of competition to promote the "best" solutions, many systems evolve which cannot communicate and share data between each other. As these systems develop it is important that standards be constructed to insure that each is compatible with the others.

14. Additional research on quality of care achieved with telemedicine is needed

Preliminary studies have indicated that the quality of care provided via telemedicine can be nearly or fully equal to that of conventional delivery systems. Additional research is needed, however, to fully evaluate quality. Federal and state agencies responsible for certifying and reimbursing healthcare costs should actively engage in dialogue with investigators to identify research questions and design appropriate studies. As with other important biomedical research questions funds should be allocated for this research.

15. With the advent of advanced telecommunications technologies, and the single national examination for medical licensure, current state-specific licensing should be reexamined

It is anticipated that most telemedicine will be intrastate in which medical licensure issues are surmountable. As provider networks evolve, however, many will appropriately cross state lines. State-by-state medical licensing significantly impedes this development. With the advent of advanced telecommunications technologies, and a single national medical licensure examination, alternatives to state-specific licensing should be examined.

16. Jurisdictional issues related to malpractice and liability must be examined if telemedicine is to achieve maximum impact on improved access to healthcare

Currently, it is unclear where liability falls when two or more practitioners cooperate on a medical problem using telemedicine. This issue should be addressed and resolved.

17. Confidentiality with respect to medical records does not appear to be any greater a problem during telemedicine than with other consultative practices

All forms of communication, from verbal to full-motion videocommunication, provide opportunities for breeches in confidentiality. Systems are available, however, to adequately insure confidentiality as long as they are properly used by the responsible individuals. Although there are unique problems during telemedicine, these problems are surmountable and should not pose a barrier to greater use of telemedicine.

Summary

The partnerships to make telemedicine work include the patient, the health care team, local, regional and long-distance carriers, and a supportive political and regulatory community. The weakest link in this partnership is patient understanding and consumer advocacy. The focus for telemedicine should be on access, but the means to deliver care have not been clearly elucidated. Educational efforts must be undertaken to lay out the realities of the present day marketplace and the potential that exists for more fully integrated programs to bring better health to each citizen. New technology that can be produced and deployed cheaply and effectively to meet economic performance standards will deliver the promise of telemedicine to health system reform.

References

1. Herbjorg Valvag: *Applied Telemedicine*, Tromso, Norway, Norwegian Telecom Research; 1992.

2. Preston J, Brown FW, Hartley B: Using telemedicine to improve health care in distant areas. *Hosp Comm Psych* 1992;43(1):25-32.

3. Watson DS: Telemedicine. *Med J Australia* 1989;151:62-71.

4. Michaels E: Telemedicine: The best is yet to come, experts say. *Canadian Med Assn J* 1989;141:612-614.

5. House M, Keough E, Hillman D, et al: Into Africa: The telemedicine links between Canada, Kenya and Uganda. *Canadian Med Assn J* 1987;136:398-400.

6. Lindsay EA, Davis DA, Fallis F, Willison DB, Biggar J: Continuing education through telemedicine for Ontario. *Canadian Med Assn J* 1987;137:503-506.

7. Dongier M, Tempier R, Lalinec-Michaud M, Meunier D: Telepsychiatry: Psychiatric consultation through two-way television. A controlled study. *Canadian J Psych* 1986;31:32-34.

8. Allen A, Cox C, Calvina T: Telemedicine in Kansas. *Kansas Medicine* 1993;93:323-325.

9. Ackerman LV, Gitlin JN: ACR-NEMA Digital imaging communication standard: Demonstration at RSNA '92 InfoRAD. *Radiology* 1992;Nov; 185(2):394.

10. Scott WW,Jr., Rosenbaum JE, Ackerman SJ, et al: Subtle orthopedic fractures: Teleradiology workstation versus film interpretation. *Radiology* 1993;June; 187(3):811-815.

11. Ackerman SJ, Gitlin JN, Gayler RW, Flagle CD, Bryan RN: Receiver operating characteristic analysis of fracture and pneumonia detection: Comparison of laser-digitized workstation images and conventional analog radiographs. *Radiology* 1993;Jan; 186(1):263-268.

12. Gitlin JN,Professor: The ACR-NEMA standard for medical image communication. Norwegian Telecom Research; Tromso, Norway; May 20-22. *First International Conference on Medical Aspects of Telemecine* 1993;56.(Abstract)

13. Wondrow MA, Wegwerth PJ, Mitchell MP, Gilbert BK: A study of medical image data compression. *SMPTE Journal* 1993;January:9-13.

14. Martinez R,Ph.D.: Design of global communications networks for telemedicine applications. Norwegian Telecom Research; Tromso, Norway; May 20-22. *First International Conference on Medical Aspects of Telemecine* 1993;33.(Abstract)

15. Weinstein RS, Bloom KJ, Rozek LS: Telepathology. Long-distance diagnosis. *Am J Clin Pathol* 1989;April; 91(4 suppl 1):S39-S42.

16. Krupinski EA,Ph.D.: Technology assessment of medical video images. Norwegian Telecom Research; Tromso, Norway; May 20-22. *First International Conference on Medical Aspects of Telemedicine* 1993;49.(Abstract)

17. Weinstein RS,M.D.: Static versus dynamic imaging in telepathology. Norwegian Telecom Research; Tromso, Norway; May 20-22. *First International Conference on Medical Aspects of Telemedicine* 1993;49.(Abstract)

18. Murphy RL, Block P, Bird KT, Yurchak T: Accuracy of ascultation by microwave. *Chest* 1973;63(4); April:578-581.

Mr. HAYES. Thank you very much.
Colonel Gomez, please.

STATEMENT OF DR. EDWARD GOMEZ, M.D., F.A.C.S., LTC, MEDICAL CORPS, U.S. ARMY, CHIEF, PERIPHERAL VASCULAR SURGERY, WALTER REED MEDICAL CENTER, WASHINGTON, DC

Dr. GOMEZ. Congressman Hayes, Congresswoman Morella, thank you very much for inviting us to participate in this very important hearing. I would like to present my comments and reflect very much the comments of Dr. Sanders and Dr. Tangalos, and we have shared the same concerns and have some very innovative experience that we would like to share with everyone.

I would like to spend a few moments going over our most recent experience in terms of a humanitarian effort as part of Operation Restore Hope, and then close with some of our new directives within DOD.

May I have the first slide?

What I would like to start off with first is the project that we have just completed called Remote Clinical Communication System which provides our physicians in the field with a new and integrated method of medical consultation incorporating our latest technological advantages. It gives us almost instant access to Walter Reed from these remote mobile facilities.

In December of 1992, the Surgeon General of the Army, Lieutenant General Alcide LaNoue, directed a task force to determine the best clinical and technical approach in order to provide immediate medical consultative services on a worldwide basis.

All available current technology for communications were carefully reviewed and the project was deployed as part of the humanitarian effort of Operation Restore Hope.

Previous experience following the Armenian earthquake by a joint effort between the Soviet Union and NASA demonstrated the feasibility of international telemedicine communication.

Again, as Dr. Sanders has mentioned to you, we based our system off off-the-shelf technology, utilizing computers, software, portable high-speed satellite communications and importantly, digital photography. It provided digital transmission of the information to include both audio and video data.

The digital information included high resolution medical images which I will give you examples of. In designing the system, the following factors were critical: It was focused on physician use, that is, physician to physician contact for the remote hospital to the medical center.

A system with ease of use and more importantly ease of access was a key feature. Training with a selected platform was minimal, as was experienced by Dr. Sanders at the Medical College or Georgia.

Access to the equipment is easy. In addition, the system is designed to be consultative in nature and thus be able to access the multiple medical disciplines and integrate with the established databases.

At Walter Reed, it was linked to both MEDLINE and also through CHCS, which is our health computer system for DOD. We looked also at the advantages and disadvantages of both systems. Digital systems have certain advantages which included high-resolution still images, data storage and very important to us was maintenance of patient confidentiality, an issue that will probably be discussed at length in this hearing.

It also provided us with a user friendly platform and more importantly kept our costs down. The digital system was adapted as the backbone for image information.

Conceptually, this was accomplished with remote access computing using small portable computers with high-speed modems and satellite communications. The field computer that was selected was, again, lightweight, portable, and had a wealth of software packages built into it that allowed the physician to have essentially a work station. The digital system was based on a digital camera that allowed us to have a digital image captured without having to do the transfer from analog to digital back to analog, and this was stored—images were taken and stored.

The images are excellent for consultative purposes and its primary application has been speed and distance. As you see here, the entire package is lightweight and it can be deployed with a mobile hospital. The satellite system used for Somalia was based on the Worldwide International Maritime Satellite System.

For the medical center, that is at Walter Reed, the system is a little more extensive and capable of both data storage and expansion. The computer system has graphic enhancement capabilities that is based on an easy to learn access approach. The computer incorporates an optical disk drive for image storage, high resolution color printers allowing the media printing for electronic photograph without the need of a dark room and a communications package for both commercial line and INMARSAT communications.

An important feature of our system though was the development and establishment of telemedicine service, and this is a full-time, 24 hour on-call system. The physicians assigned to the telemedicine service are instructed on the use of the equipment, the communication systems, preparations of the graphic data and finally, completion of consultations received from Somalia. This full response system, despite time zone differences, remain the most important factor for the success of the telemedicine concept.

Our system works in the following scenario: A physician in the field encounters a difficult medical problem and seeks consultation. The physician is able to prepare a written profile on the patient's history and physical examination, and he obtains an electronic still photograph with the use of a computerized digital camera to illustrate the problem.

These images and clinical information are downloaded by the portable computer. The information is then transmitted by satellite or commercial line to Walter Reed. Physicians supporting the telemedicine service review the clinical information and images. Following their assessment, the physicians can provide additional expert medical information to the physicians in the field either by cellular phone or response with computer communication systems.

Our first deployment for this system was with the United States Army's 86th Evacuation Hospital. This is a 104-bed hospital that was deployed as part of Operation Restore Hope. We deployed this

81-951 O - 94 - 4

system in February of 1993. This hospital is represented with several surgical and medical specialties to include thoracic surgery, maxillofacial surgery and neurosurgery, specialties that can be seen in a rather advanced deployment hospital.

The system was later used by other replacement combat support hospitals to include the 42nd Combat Support Hospital and the 46th Combat Support Hospital.

During this deployment, a variety of consults were received from Somalia and the following are clinical examples. These are all digital images that were sent from Somalia and it sort of illustrates the quality of images we were receiving. It also illustrates the variety of patients that we were consulted further.

This unfortunately is a seven year old boy who presented there, Somali civilian with injuries. Interesting, this consult was presented to plastic surgery who managed his care over 8,000 miles away.

This is a young Marine who had a fragment wound to the eye with a cornea abrasion. As you can see, the high definition image allowed us to manage his wound in the field.

This is another civilian injury that was presented to us who had disruption of both the vein and the artery, and again our specialists at Walter Reed were able to assist in the postoperative management of this particular patient.

Here is a United Nations soldier who, unfortunately, sustained this very extensive injury, and we can get both the clinical images and the X-rays and his management with hand surgery was accomplished over this distance, and finally this is another young Somali girl who presented with a non-union of her lower extremity, and this consultation was carried on utilizing the specialists at Walter Reed.

And then finally the system was deployed also to Zagreb, Croatia and Macedonia as part of other United Nations' efforts and this is a young United Nations soldier presenting with a left lower lung pneumonia. This smear shows a fungus and management was coordinated with the pulmonary specialists at Walter Reed.

And then this final case that I have for you to illustrate the spectrum of consults that we received from these countries, this is another United Nations soldier who had a fragment wound as shown by the arrows here in his left ventricle, and this was an electrocardiogram that was sent to the cardiothoracic surgeons at Walter Reed for additional consultation.

If we look at Somalia though, the overall majority of consults were to the medical specialists, such a dermatology, infectious disease and ophthalmology. Specialists are not usually deployed with an evacuation hospital. This represents an important impact on management on noncombat injuries, particularly in a humanitarian effort such as Operation Restore Hope.

The results of our experience are as follows: This represents the first extended use of telemedicine for humanitarian purposes incorporating digital images and satellite communication. This system was functional for 13 months, from the period of February 1993 through March of this year by three individual hospitals.

The important lessons that we learned from this project was the importance of physician training, input by the end user during the development and design, the establishment of a flexible, reliable work station with multiple capabilities to access established databases and also communications systems such as Internet, storage of clinical data, and really a dedicated teleconferencing system.

Clearly there are several benefits. We did reduce our lost time. We did reduce the interval of medical expenses while awaiting definitive care, and obviously we increased the productivity of our physicians in the field.

Furthermore, from our Somali experience, hardware can be changed. It has to be interchangeable. We really had no difficulty with our system throughout this. As we have change though our direction, this will provide a valuable link for future system development and the continuing education of field medicine and planning for future operations.

In DOD, particularly the U.S. Army, we are interested in establishing a global military telemedicine hub being able to expand regionally to support day-to-day practice within our own medical communities, and also have applications into the civilian sector for remote areas, importantly for disaster relief, and finally, direction is being looked at to explore in the emerging communications and computer imagining technologies.

Under the direction of the United States Army Medical Department Telemedicine Program at Fort Detrick, they are looking at providing applications of both peacetime and wartime, providing this specialty care as far forward as possible while reducing deployment requirements and all in order to follow the guidelines set by the President, that is, establish an international information infrastructure to promote universal health access.

Thank you.

[The prepared statement of Edward Gomez, M.D., F.A.C.S. follows:]

Walter Reed Army Medical Center

Telemedicine Service

US Army Medical Research, Development, Acquisitions and Logistics Command

Telemedicine Project Office

Walter Reed Army Medical Center and the U. S. Army Medical Research, Development, Acquisition and Logistics Command combines the Medical Research and Development Command (USAMRDAL), Medical Materiel Agency (USAMMA) and Health Facilities Planning Agency (USAHFPA) into a major subordinate command of the provisional Army Medical Command (MEDCOM).

USAMRDAL has undertaken research and development initiatives to establish telemedicine in military operations in peacetime and war. Telemedicine includes telemonitoring, telementoring, teleconsulting, and, in the future, telesurgery. It also encompasses digital medical records and the "wireless" hospital. The Army Medical Department (AMEDD) has identified clear benefits which will be realized if telemedicine is adopted; at the current time, these benefits are qualitative not quantitative. The AMEDD has also developed preliminary estimates of costs primarily, for subsystems and components. The AMEDD is the best suited of the various services to undertake this research and "Proof of Principle" development for the following reasons:

- The Army medical community faces the most difficult changes because it takes a much larger percentage of its medical community to the wartime theatre and it operates in a more difficult environment once there.

- Army medical units are typically the first deployment in both wartime and in operations other than war.

- Advances in telemedicine will allow the Army to deploy full capability with less structure to the area of operations through improved use of both the residual medical capability which remains in major fixed medical hospitals and the deployed medical forces.

- The resultant reduction in the in-theatre infrastructure (numbers of soldiers and tons of medical equipment) obtained by this improved telemedicine capability allows an improved tooth-to-tail ratio within theatre and the ability to deploy more combat assets with a given amount of lift, while still providing full medical support to the deployed personnel.

- When deployed to the are of operations, be that overseas or within the United States, the Army tactical medical units typically operate in an austere environment. Procedures and technology that work in this most challenging environment can be utilized by any of the other medical providers.

- Medical care in a tactical environment is often provided by medical professionals, at all levels from corpsman to neurosurgeon, who because of the dispersion of assets across the battlefield must deliver that care without the ability to seek assistance from peers or mentors.

- Legislative action two years ago now allows the National Guard to provide in-service medical treatment to medically underserviced areas as part of its ongoing training. The telemedicine initiatives would allow the Guard to link back to major medical resources such as Walter Reed Army Medical Center, thus improving the quality of medical services available in rural or urban areas at the same time Guard personnel are being mentored by the finest physicians in the country.

- This Telemedicine program promotes the Clinton administration's goal of universal equal access to quality care as well as providing another tangible use of the emerging National Information Infrastructure.

Appendix
Telemedicine Vision of the Future
Walter Reed Army Medical Center

The Remote Clinical Communications System (RCCS) discussed by Dr. Gomez represents an initial foray into telemedicine at Walter Reed Army Medical Center. Analysis of initial patient care and cost/benefit data from the telemedicine projects in Somalia, Croatia and Macedonia indicates that teleconsulting (a form of on-site sub-specialty care enabled by telecommunications) and telementoring (a form of on-the-job medical tutoring from a remote location) have potential for more extensive applications. Of particular interest is the potential for direct clinical support in day-to-day health care practice in both the civilian and military communities, especially in remote areas where sub-specialty consultation normally requires significant travel by either the patient or the physician consultant. Our cost/benefit study suggests that telemedicine can reduce costs associated with physician travel and patient evacuation while improving health care provided regionally, as well as in remote locations. Therefore, further investment in telemedicine technology is warranted.

While we intend to enhance and expand Walter Reed's role as a center for world-wide telemedicine support for deployed U.S. and U.N. forces, we also intend to expand our telemedicine capabilities to support day-to-day military health care within our assigned Department of Defense and Army health care regions. This service can be expanded to include civilian telemedicine support to remote areas where other consultation support is not yet available or in support of disaster relief. Walter Reed's telemedicine services could be offered directly by the Department of Defense or through the Veterans' Administration; the Indian Health Services; or through the State Department for U.N. Trust Territories, foreign military services, or developing nations where indigenous sub-specialty consultation is not available.

Walter Reed's telemedicine expansion plans require integration of existing clinical information systems with ongoing telemedicine projects within both the military and civilian communities. Expanded telemedicine capabilities will require exploitation of new technologies such as acquisition and delivery of very high resolution, full-motion video digital imaging at the physician's desk-top computer and connection to high performance data communications networks which are emerging as a result of the President's national data highway initiative. In addition to ongoing telemedicine projects in radiology, pathology, dermatology, and anatomy; potential applications exist in preventive medicine and public health services such as disease surveillance, epidemiologic investigations and biomedical engineering. Whatever the application, Walter Reed will continue to explore development of telemedicine-based practice as a method of saving resources while improving health care delivery.

Remote Global Telemedicine

Experience during Operation Restore Hope

A
Joint
Office of the Army Surgeon General
and
Walter Reed Army Medical Center
Project

INTRODUCTION

This project named Remote Clinical Communication System provides the physicians in the field with a new and integrated method of consultation incorporating the latest technological advances in data and image transfer. It gives almost instant access to the medical center from the mobile remote facilities.

BACKGROUND

In December of 1992, the Surgeon General of the Army, Lieutenant General Alcide LaNoue, directed a task force to determine the best clinical and technical approach in order to provide immediate medical consultative services on a worldwide basis. All available current technology for communications were carefully reviewed. The project was deployed as part of the humanitarian effort of Operation Restore Hope.

Previous experience following the Armenian earthquake by a joint effort between the Soviet Union and NASA demonstrated the feasibility of the international telemedicine communication.

DESIGN

This system is based on "off-the-shelf" computers, software, portable high speed satellite telecommunications and digital photography. It provides digital transmission of information to include both audio and video data. The digital information includes high resolution medical images.

In designing the system, the following factors are critical. It is focused on physician use; that is, physician to physician contact, from the remote hospital to the medical center. A system with ease of use and more importantly, ease of access is the key feature. Training with the selected platform is minimal. Access to the equipment is easy. In addition, the system is designed to be consultative in nature, to reach multiple medical disciplines and to integrate with the established databases. At Walter Reed, it was linked to both MEDLINE, through the MEDLARS at the National Library of Medicine and through CHCS, the health computer system for the Department of Defense.

Both analog and digital systems were reviewed with advantages and disadvantages of respective technologies compared. Digital systems have several advantages including high resolution still images, data storage, maintenance of patient confidentiality, user friendly platform and most importantly low commercial cost and available. The digital system was adapted as the backbone for image information

This conceptual approach is accomplished with remote access computing using small compact portable computers with high speed modems and satellite communications for the transfer of both clinical data and images.

TECHNICAL FEATURES

REMOTE SITE REQUIREMENTS

The field computer system is a light, portable laptop system with built-in modems and multiple software packages giving the physician a wealth of computing power including a designed database, word-processing, communication package and graphic programs. The overall response has been is that indeed it is easy to learn, is dependable and portable.

The digital camera is based on the latest technology capable of capturing a high resolution digital medical image and storing it on a built-in hard disk drive. The color images are excellent for consultative purposes and its primary application has been speed and distance. The entire package deployed to the mobile hospital is light weight and portable.

The satellite communications used for Somalia is based on the Worldwide International Maritime Satellite System, INMARSAT.

MEDICAL CENTER SYSTEM

For the medical center, the system is more extensive and capable of data storage and expansion. The computer system has graphic enhancement capabilities and also based on the easy to learn and access approach. The computer incorporates an optical disk drive for image storage, a high resolution color printer allowing immediate printing of the electronic photographs without the need of a dark room, a communications package both for commercial line and INMARSAT communications.

TELEMEDICINE SERVICE

The key important factor is the establishment of a Telemedicine Service, a full-time, 24 hour on-call system . The physicians were instructed on the use of the equipment, communications systems, preparation of graphic data and finally the completion of the consultations received from Somalia. This full response system despite time zone differences remains the most important factor for the success of the TeleMedicine concept.

EXAMPLE

This system works similar to the following scenario. A physician is the field encounters a difficult medical problem and seeks consultation. The physician is able to prepare a written profile on the patient's history and physical examination and obtains an electronic still photograph with the use of a computerized digital camera to illustrate the problem. These images and clinical information are downloaded by portable computer. The information is then transmitted by satellite or commercial lines to Walter Reed. Physicians supporting the TeleMedicine review the clinical information and high quality computer generated transmitted images. Following their assessment, the physicians provide addition expert medical information to the physician in the field either by cellular phone or response with the computer communication system.

SOMALIA EXPERIENCE

The system was initially deployed to the US Army's 86th Evacuation Hospital, a 104 bed hospital. This hospital was represented with several surgical and medical specialties to include Thoracic Surgery, Maxillofacial Surgery and Neurosurgery, specialties representative of a community hospital. This system was later used by other replacement combat support hospitals to include the 42nd Combat Support Hospital and the 46th Combat Support Hospital. During this deployment, a variety of consults were received from Somalia, to several medical specialties such as Dermatology, Infectious Disease and Ophthalmology. This represented an important impact in the management of non-combat injuries, particularly in a humanitarian effort such as Operation Restore Hope.

CONCLUSIONS

This Remote Telemedicine Project represents the first extended use of Telemedicine for humanitarian purposes incorporating digital images and satellite communications. This system was used for 13 months from February 1993 through March 1994 by three separate military hospitals. Important features included the enhancement of patient care, ease of access and use of the system by the field physician, the ability to provide both consultative and diagnostic services, and easy medical record transfer. Important lessons, learned during this experience, included importance of physician training, input by the end-user in the development and design, and a reliable, flexible work station with multiple capabilities to include access to establish databases, storage of clinical data and images, and rarely a dedicated teleconferencing system.

Furthermore, from the Somalia experience, current hardware systems deployed were reliable with no downtime despite unfriendly environmental conditions. Software systems, incorporated into the workstation were indeed valid. The graphics program served as a backbone of the system. The database maintained the medical record and allowed for assessment of clinical information. This will provide a valuable link for future system development, the continuing education of field medicine and planning for future applications.

The system was later deployed to Zagreb, Croatia and Landstuhl, Germany as part of other important United Nations efforts.

REMOTE CLINICAL CONSULTATION SYSTEM
RCCS

Submitted to: The Surgeon General
Submitted from: COL Joan T. Zajtchuk, LTC Ed Gomez, LTC Ron Propopatich, MAJ Tom Kryzer, LTC Gary Gilbert and LTC Jim O'Keiff, Walter Reed Army Medical Center

Purpose:
Present cost and benefit information developed during the alpha testing of the RCCS from the Somalia peacekeeping mission.

Definitions:

Remote Clinical Consultation System (RCCS). A system consisting of voice and digital transmission of photos, text, computer, and satellite technology to assist in diagnosis and treatment of patients from around the world.

Fixed Costs. Costs which remain constant regardless of changes in business activity.

Variable Costs. Costs which tend to vary with changes in business activity.

Personnel Costs. Costs outlined below do not include personnel cost.

Costs:

Fixed Costs: The system is a combination of the following components:

Hardware

o Computers - A combination of laptop and PC based systems.

o Image capturing equipment - Fax, Kodak Digital Camera System (DCS) mounted on Nikon single lens reflex camera body.

o Output Devices - Color monitors, Kodak digital color pictures, fax machines, and laser printers.

Communication Interface: 2400/9600 bps modems

Communication Medium Portable International Maritime Satellite (IMS) unit uplink to COMSAT satellite and commercial telecommunication lines.

REMOTE CLINICAL CONSULTATION SYSTEM
RCCS

Hardware Description: The following equipment is required at the deployed medical treatment site and the fixed medical treatment facility.

FLY AWAY PACKAGE

Description	Cost per Item
PowerBook Duo 230 120/4	$2,743
Macintosh Duo Dock	$997
Apple Extended Keyboard II	$147
Macintosh 14" Color Display	$628
RasterOps 24STV Frame Grabber	$815
Camera	$8,342
Fax Machine	$1,700
Modem	$800
Adobe PhotoShop 2.0	$528
Microsoft Word	$278
Smartcom	$83
MAGNAPHONE Satellite Transmitter	$36,000
Total Fixed Cost per Unit	$53,061
Total Cost for Deployable unit (2 units required for redundancy)	$106,122

Fixed Medical Treatment Facility Equipment

Description	Cost per Item
QUADRA 950 230/8 CPU	$5,796
CENTRIS CPU	$3,200
Apple 21" Color Monitor	$3,469
Apple 14" Color Monitor	$628
Apple Extended Keyboard II (2 each)	$147
Memory Expansion (2 each)	$1,200
Kodak Color Photo Printer,	$16,000
Camera	$8,342
Stylewriter Printer	$300
Modem	$800
Adobe PhotoShop 2.0	$528
Microsoft Word	$278
Smartcom	$83
Total WRAMC Equipment	$42,289

Total Fixed Costs ***$148,411***

If a 3 year usable life is used to depreciate this equipment, the annual expense for the fixed cost equals *$49,169/year.*

REMOTE CLINICAL CONSULTATION SYSTEM
RCCS

Variable Costs

Components

- Communications Expense (satellite time per/minute)
- Supplies
- Utilities

Discussion: Development of variable cost of telemedicine consult per patient. The following variable cost resources per consultant are projected:

Communication Expense. Per minute expense is $5.34. An average consult requires the transmission of:		
2 photo images @ 15 minutes/ image	$160.20	
1 faxed document @ 5 minutes/fax	$26.70	
1 phoncon @ 5 minutes/discussion	$26.70	
Average Communication per consult		**$218.94**
Supply Costs (per consult):		
Fax document expenses	$.10	
Miscellaneous expenses	$.25	
Color Printer costs:$4.00/image X 2 images	$8.00	
Average Supply Cost (per consult):		**$8.35**
Utilities Expenses are insignificant:	$ .00	
Total Average Variable Cost/ Consult:		**$227.29**

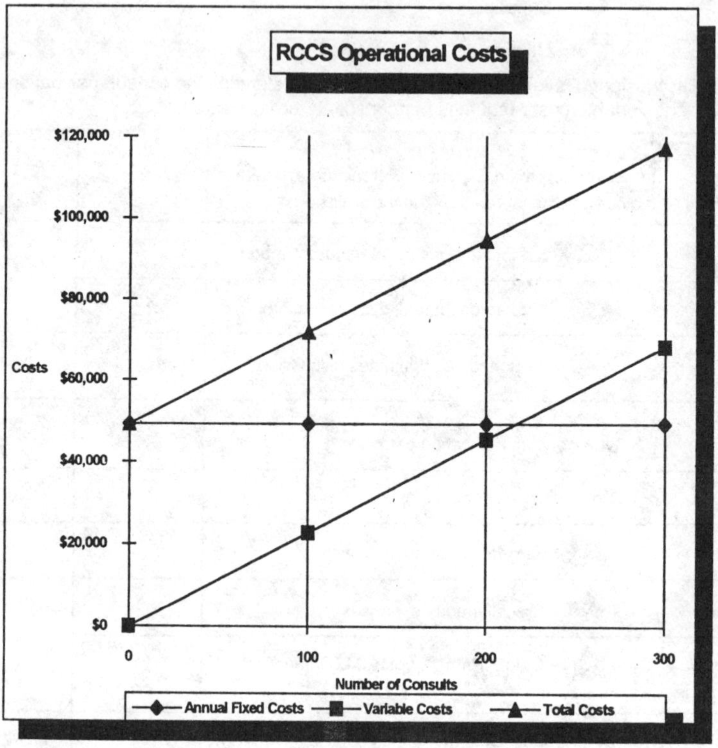
RCCS Operational Costs
$120,000
$100,000
$80,000
$60,000
$40,000
$20,000
$0
Costs
0
100
200
300
Number of Consults
Annual Fixed Costs
Variable Costs
Total Costs

Benefit Determination

Discussion.

✈ This analysis concentrates on the tangible, as opposed to intangible, benefits of the RCCS. This analysis will focus on the potential savings of preventing the evacuation of a soldier from a theater of operations, rather than attempting to quantify the value of the collegial aspects of the RCCS.

✈ Our hypothesis to calculate cost avoidance is based on 202 cases for air evacuation from Somalia between February and March 1993. At least 15% of patients were returned to their primary duty station after evacuation from Landstuhl Army Regional Medical Center (LARMC). Ten percent of patients were evacuated to CONUS. It appeared that even with a minor diagnosis that the final destination of the patient was CONUS. It is presumed that approximately 25% of patients evacuated from the theater may have avoided air evacuation by employing RCCS technology. We then used this data to extrapolate cost avoidance for the period February through December 1993.

✈ The data upon which this analysis is constructed is based on the Operation Restore Hope (February through December 1993) experience. Without additional research,.conclusions drawn are preliminary and cannot be applied to other than peacekeeping missions.

✈ The report will not address the following issues:

■ Some air evac patients were admitted from an outpatient status. Telemedicine may have benefited this group of patients. To get a more accurate picture of the need to evacuate, more stringent evacuation policies are required.

■ Also in the cost avoidance computations the cost of actual evacuation, ie airframe expenses were not included.

Facts:

✈ During the period February through December 1993, 450 patients were regulated/evacuated from Somalia.

✈ The average evacuation rate = 41soldiers/month.

✈ The size of the US Force on the ground in Somalia during the period was approximately 14,000 soldiers.

✈ Given the above facts, the air evacuation rate per month for 1,000 soldiers supported = 2.9 evacuations/month.

REMOTE CLINICAL CONSULTATION SYSTEM
RCCS

Conclusions: After reviewing 202 air evacuations from Somalia, LTC Gomez and MAJ Kryzer, concluded the following:

✈ 10% of the patients regulated from Somalia to LARMC were returned to duty.

✈ The evacuated patients who were returned to duty from LARMC could have been treated in Somalia.

✈ Patients evacuated to LARMC and subsequently returned to duty in Somalia would lose 7 duty days, or $672 in payroll expense. Transportation costs were not calculated due to the fact that these flight are not totally dependent on a particular patient is or not scheduled.

✈ 15% of the patients evacuated from Somalia and subsequently moved to CONUS could have been treated in Somalia. We were not able to discern whether some of these patients could have been returned from LARMC.

✈ Soldiers evacuated from Somalia to CONUS require a replacement. The time necessary to have the replacement to the unit in Somalia would be 30 days. The payroll expense.would be $2,880

✈ The average grade for an evacuated soldier was SGT, with an annual salary of approximately $35,000. Daily salary cost = $96.

✈ A total of 25% of the patients regulated could have been treated in Somalia by utilizing the RCCS.

✈ The financial impact of the dimunation of unit effectiveness due to preventable medical evacuations is not estimated.

Analysis: The following three graphs display the economics involved in this analysis

→ This first chart reflects the expected number of patients requiring evacuation based on the extrapolation of the Somalia experience.

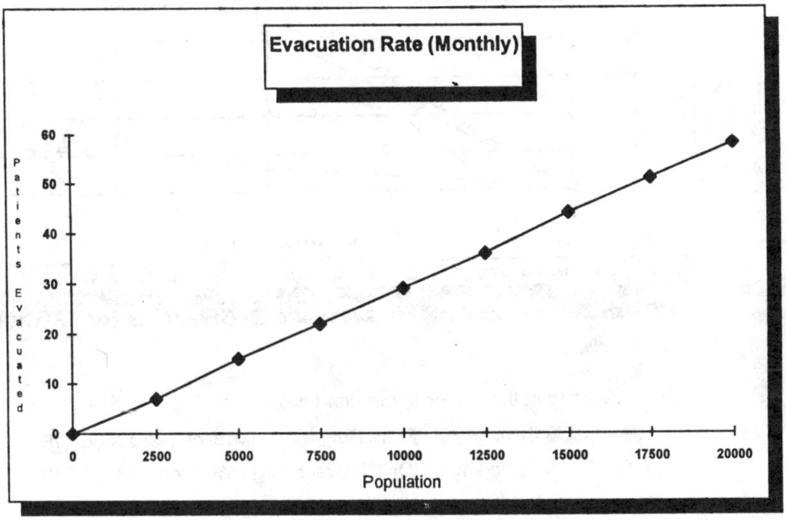

REMOTE CLINICAL CONSULTATION SYSTEM
RCCS

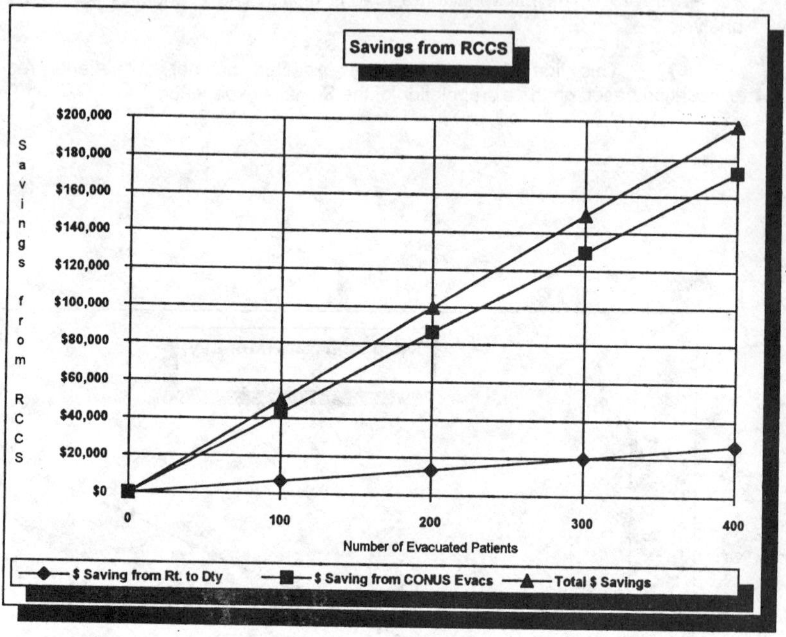

→ A recap of the figures in this chart are:

- ◆ $ Savings from Rt. to Duty = (10% of evacs X $672/RTD),
- ■ $ Saving from CONUS Evacs = (15% of evacs X $2,880/CONUS)
- ▲ Total Savings is the combination of the above

→ This chart depicts the savings to be accrued by employing RCCS with the intent of reducing the cost associated with the personnel expenses incurred with a preventable evacuation.

REMOTE CLINICAL CONSULTATION SYSTEM
RCCS

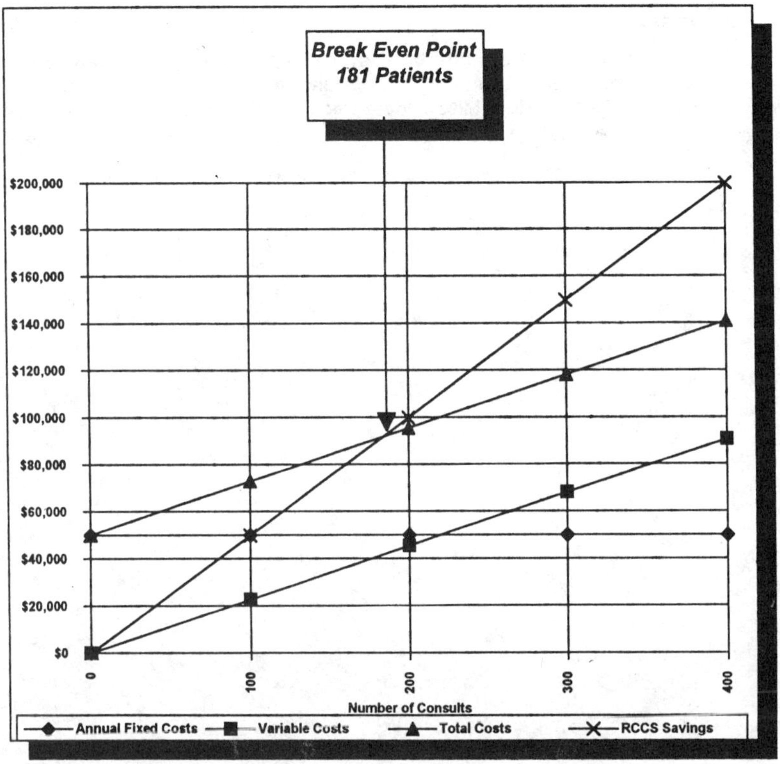

Break Even Point = (Fixed Costs + (Variable Costs * # of Evacs)) -RCCS Cost Savings.

✈ The last chart clearly reveals the break even point associated with the employment of this technology. The actual break even point is 181 patients.

✈ If the cost associated with the airframes required to support these evacuations was included, the break even point would drop precipitously.

REMOTE CLINICAL CONSULTATION SYSTEM
RCCS

Summary.

✈ In the Somalia theater the break even analysis reveals that as few as 181 consults annually can provide sufficient cost avoidance to support the cost associated with a RCCS. The Restore Hope Mission data predicts that a 5,000 person force would generate 181 consults in a year.

✈ This study should serve as a proposal for a more definitive study.

Mr. HAYES. I want to thank you too.

I am not going to spend a great deal of time on questions, but I do want to make an observation, ask a question related to that of the previous panel.

When I was in Augusta—I also don't play golf, by the way, you can tell Mr. Rather that. When I was in Augusta on the hearing involving an entirely different issue and had an opportunity to tour your site, one of the things that I remembered most vividly was the cost comparison concept of moving folks in correctional institutions, the fact that you have to have guards go with them, high security, very high and expensive movement, made this kind of technology unbelievably valuable in that instance to the correctional system. I am going to imagine that that has been borne out by further experience.

I noticed it was in your chart earlier, and I would also like to know how the State of Georgia, if the State of Georgia is keeping track of its cost comparativeness as well as its delivery of service so that it might be of use as a model in other jurisdictions, other States, and other cities. Dr. Sanders.

Dr. JAY SANDERS. The experience in the correctional institution to date has shown that 90 percent of the prisoners are—they like to call them inmates, that used to have to be transferred, are now kept at the local site. Based upon these early results, they plan to do a State-wide expansion into corrections.

The issue of the economic impact, not only in corrections, but in rural and in the—those people who are socioeconomically isolated, will be done now with the expansion to the 60 sites. We are undertaking a very comprehensive State-wide evaluation, not only of the economics and the technology and the quality, but also the psychological impact on both physician and patient.

So I will be able, hopefully within two to three years, to be a lot more definitive and a lot more certain about the data that I can provide.

We do have data from the past. There have been telemedicine initiatives that have been in existence for about 27 years. One of the original ones, where I first came in contact with telemedicine, was at the Massachusetts General Hospital in Boston back in 1967 when I was a resident, and there have been studies over the years which have addressed the issues of quality, economics, technology and psychological impact. Most of these studies have been quite positive.

Mr. HAYES. That is very interesting. I am also curious and ask any of you, we have invited you here today, I think it is very useful. I also think that having listened to the—and seen the things that you have told us and had some of the visuals that go with it, that you ought to well consider inviting yourselves to things like the National Conference of Governors that was here not long ago.

I would think that that opportunity, and opportunities like that, I know it is taking away from your valuable time, would be extremely well received and allow people who work in different levels of State government to see what is going on in the military, out of the military, Walter Reed, over at Mayo, and of course an entire State network like Georgia, and would say anyway we could assist that, we would be delighted to do so because there are just an enormous number of people who ought to have the benefit of seeing what we saw today, and I want to thank you again for your presentations. I will turn this over to Ms. Morella.

Mrs. MORELLA. Thank you. I want to thank you also. Maybe that could be done, Mr. Chairman, through telecommunication. You could be where you are and also before the Governors Conference.

I appreciated very much your oral testimony, the visual and the work that has gone on to make that all possible.

Dr. Sanders, I was also interested in the fact that correctional institutions could utilize keeping people where they are. I found it very interesting that you talked about it being like off-the-shelf technology so when we talk about technology being so expensive as one of the handicaps, you are saying you could use it for ordinary information that specialists have and just bring it to the homes of rural communities.

And you demonstrated the fact that you would save money for hospitals, your doctor or your nurse practitioner would be there with the patients. Are you trying to point out that actually you save money starting off now with telemedicine in its basic form?

Would you like to explain that? Because I found that to be something that seemed to emerge from your testimony.

Dr. JAY SANDERS. Yes. As a matter of fact, there are two sides to that coin. Dr. Smits hit on it also. Back in 1973, we had a $1.2 million grant from the National Science Foundation to study telemedicine, and one of the areas that we were asked to look at was the economics of the system. And I think the results that we got then would be totally applicable to my response to your question.

We found that the per-patient cost of care over telemedicine was less than if we had brought the patient into the facility. But the overall cost of care of the entire system was higher. The reason for that was the system was successful. It did improve access to care and, therefore, all the people who had been previously disenfranchised from the health care system that now could be seen and have that access, the volume was higher than the per-patient cost decrease.

I think whether we are talking telemedicine or any health care initiative, I think we had better realize that if it works, the people who have not had access to the care, whether rural communities or in the inner city, now when they have access to care, that volume may actually drive up the cost for four to six years until some of the preventive health care initiatives and perhaps some of the home health care telemedicine initiatives take on to avoid repeat hospitalizations.

Mrs. MORELLA. We have thought in State legislatures and the Federal Congress about home medicare and the idea that this would keep people from nursing homes. But the point is, you would need so much because more people would need home health care and more people that need nursing homes. So it is not really the equipment that is that expensive; it is the expansion.

Dr. JAY SANDERS. Yes. The average cost of the system when we first put that first remote site November 1991, that system cost $200,000. Today that system costs approximately $130,000. What we are seeing is an inverse relationship between the improvement in the technology and the cost of the technology.

Secondly, if I increased the bed census of a rural hospital in Georgia by a single patient, change their bed census from 25 patients per day per year to 26 patients per day per year, that nets out to that rural hospital administrator to $150,000 a year net cash flow. So a single patient cap more than pays for putting in the system.

Mrs. MORELLA. Do you have a way of communicating this to all the major hospitals in the country? Do they know about this so they can jump on the bandwagon?

Dr. JAY SANDERS. Those of us sitting on the panel I know are being called on a daily basis and being asked how do we do this. We find a lot of major academic institutions who have awakened and realized that there is a moat that has been built around their institution that they haven't built but the outside world has, that a way for them to sustain their market, a way for them to expand their market is with the introduction of this type of telecommunication network.

Dr. TANGALOS. One thing concerning the cost, we talked about the hardware costs but there are significant costs in connectivity. I tried to get at some of that with the testimony. With regard to the policy issues that face Congress, we have tremendous expenses in making connections work. Whether it be local, regional Bell operating companies, or cable networks, most of the telemedicine programs are suffering under the expense to make these linkages work, and we don't have a cooperative communications policy going on right now.

We have very disparate policies and with each line change, with each passing off of service, there is an extra expense and an extra problem related to that. If you talk to other groups that are involved, like the West Virginia project, it is the cost of the services to make the connections that prohibit a lot of the service. That is why you hear repeatedly the idea to use these services for multifunctional activities, not just medical services, but link them to distance learning and economic redevelopment. That brings down the costs of connectivity.

There is one other thing that I would like to touch upon with regard—we say that managed care is the easy way to find the answer, that you leave it up to a managed care system and they will do that. We have placed undue burden in telemedicine upon managed care in that they have to consider a whole variety of other expenses that we don't consider in the fee-for-service environment, and it puts them at a disadvantage, whereas managed care might have to consider the driving cost to keep the patient at home or all the down time. And to be competitive, managed care has to go head to head similarly with the fee-for-service environment.

Right now, fee-for-service doesn't consider how long it may take a patient to get 300 miles or how many days are lost. We ask telemedicine networks to do that automatically, but we have to include in that discussion how much money will be saved on the one side that the other group is not accountable for at all.

Mrs. MORELLA. That gets into the results evaluation too. Is there a way of measuring as many managed care facilities?

Dr. TANGALOS. I think the programs that come on line and go forward need to be outcome measures and good economic measures put into that. HCFA has one of the projects going on with Denver right now. It was my responsibility in October with the Office of Rural Health Policy to look at outcome-based studies. There essentially aren't any.

I think as we fund projects, these projects need to be funded with the proviso that good economics and good outcome analyses be part of the research?

Mrs. MORELLA. Could outcome-based studies be in a short period of time?

Dr. TANGALOS. You can design both ways, have acute interventions and get information longitudinally, but right now, the projects haven't had the money or requirement to do that.

Mrs. MORELLA. Linking up, just the other day in Post Office, Civil Service Committee, we had somebody show us how we will be able to use our cable TV to decide what postal stamps we want to buy, what the weight is going to be. You can do catalogue shopping. You can also dial in your local doctor or whatever.

And the idea is to also develop confidence in the mind of the user without having the doctor right there close to him or her. So everything is changing. Back to the future may mean you go back to an old program, too.

Dr. TANGALOS. When we put on a program in Minnesota through AHCPR, we felt that the technology and the connectivity was there, but the true lacking knowledge base was on the consumer side right now. The consumer needs to be aware and be an advocate for what can be brought into rural environments and inner city environments.

Mrs. MORELLA. Dr. Gomez, in our area, we have a place called Uniformed Services University of Health Sciences which has been on the reinvent government termination list, I think unjustly so. Is there training and uses for the kind of telemetry, the kind of medicine that you are practicing?

Dr. GOMEZ. There is. There is a committee at the school looking at telemedicine. Telemedicine at the school has been very active with Walter Reed. They are looking at distant learning, particularly with remote sites. One of the important issues we have discussed is the physician focus—in other words, continued medical education—and the school is clearly looking at that as one very important application of telemedicine.

We send our soldiers and our physicians to remote sites. They are obviously into that professional isolation and we need to be able to break that. But the medical school is, in answer to your question, really looking at this.

Mrs. MORELLA. So we now have that on record that Dr. Gomez at Walter Reed thinks it should stay in existence.

Dr. Sanders.

Dr. JAY SANDERS. One other thing relative to the use of the information highway and the point made, that is to remember that this is an information highway and it should be used for multiple purposes. One of the things that I had on one of my slides which I failed to underline was the fact that within the next 45 days, our telemedicine communication network will be totally compatible with over 100 distance learning sites within the state of Georgia in K through 12.

With our Department of Pediatrics, we are going to go into the classroom and begin some preventive health care initiatives as a first phase. And in the second phase, we are going to begin to provide episodic care with the school nurse.

What you see in many hospital emergency rooms in this country today is the fact that the child that got sick in midday during school who was sent home goes home to a empty home because there are two working parents. When the parents get home and call the general practitioner or the pediatrician, those offices are closed. Where do they end up? Inappropriately in a hospital emergency department.

We are going to see with our telemedicine whether or not we can impact on that inappropriate use of the health care system.

Mrs. MORELLA. Dr. Sanders, you mentioned—years ago, I thought it was a brave new world. They had the "feelies." You could go to the movie theater and put your arms on the seat and railing and you could feel the emotions that were being experienced on the screen. You have developed or you have talked about a glove that will do the same thing.

Can you explain that?

Dr. JAY SANDERS. Actually, it is really a transfer of technology that has been used in other areas, in protein chemistry and particularly in the nuclear energy field where remote sensors are used to touch or to feel or to grasp. We are now expanding on that and adding some sensitivities working with Georgia Tech to actually be able to transmit the sense of touch, the sense of temperature, the sense of roughness or smoothness.

The reality is that those sensations in our own body are electrical stimuli which are transmitted threw nerve fibers. We are going to try and reproduce that same type of sensation with an electronic hand. Then the issue of, well, you can't really reach out and touch me will no longer be an issue.

Dr. GOMEZ. In the Army, there are three important projects that are going on. One is advanced war fighting. We are using telemedicine to monitor the soldier in the field and monitor the corpsman as he is managing the care.

A second very important aspect is a global grid. We are able to put a telemetry device on the soldier and be able to maintain physiologically where he is in the battlefield.

A third thing, we are looking at using a surgical technique where we can do surgery in the field with a computerized hand. You could put your hand in this device and the way you move your hand, it responds at the remote site exactly the same and you could perform surgery from a distance.

Mrs. MORELLA. Are those the things that would cost money, to be able to work on the development and sophistication of such equipment?

Dr. GOMEZ. I think they clearly have a role. That is an area of R&D that needs to be looked at. The big expense is the communications network. Establishing that seems to be the biggest expense. We have a similar experience to Dr. Sanders.

We use off-the-shelf technology and our expenses are not that high. But when we look at it, we break it down in terms of number of consults and what we charge for consults, our biggest expense happens to be our communications package.

Mrs. MORELLA. What do you know about what is happening internationally? Are there other countries that are beginning to do some work in this? Is this a competitive situation?

Dr. TANGALOS. I am not sure it is a matter of worrying about the competition. We have a cooperative arrangement with some countries and Jay and I participate in projects going on in Norway. They seem to be the most active and aggressive in Europe right now. Of interest to you are the offshore projects that American companies have now.

There are at least three that we are aware of. We hinted at the one Massachusetts General Hospital has in the Middle East and Mayo has a for-profit project in Jordan with Amman diagnostic. There are a number of projects that we have going outside the country, and in Europe there are other interests as well. They have a different competitive situation in Europe.

Take Norway, for example, very much a socialized government, only one payer for health care, only one telecommunications company as well. So their deployment is based very much on government policy decisions. And they chose back in 1989 not to close any further rural hospitals. They said this is not what we are going to do, and they devoted significant national resource to their communications industry to keep those rural physicians and those patients in the towns that they grew up in and wanted to stay in. So there are different strategies going around across the country.

Mrs. MORELLA. Is this something that we might look into in terms of cost saving?

Dr. TANGALOS. We need to look at different models for delivery of a care along these lines. The policy decisions that drive these things are different types of decision processes than we have gotten into. Whether we promote a cooperative environment or stimulate a competitive environment are issues that you will have to vote on as time goes by.

Dr. JAY SANDERS. It may turn out that telemedicine will become a very large export business for the United States. I can tell you there are many countries in the Middle East, Turkey, Russia, that are exceedingly interested in downlinking with major medical centers like Mayo, for instance, in the United States.

A single example—as a matter of fact, we recently had the dean of Moscow State University School of Medicine come to see the telemedicine system in Augusta. Russia is putting in a digital signal communication network and this would be incredibly adaptable to them.

One of the smallest countries in the world and the richest country in the world per capita, United Arab Emirates, sends approximately 4 to 5,000 of their citizens, and they have a very small citizenry, a year abroad for medical care at an average cost of $35,000 per patient. Looking at the 4,000 patients at $35,000, that is $140 million a year that they spend to send patients to Mayo to Zurich, to London and for high technology, for ultra specialists? No. For an allergist, for a dermatologist because they don't have that expertise in their country. They are very interested in downlinking with medical centers in the United States.

Dr. TANGALOS. The qualifications of the trained physicians in the Middle East are very good as they are across Europe, but the western second opinion cannot be overstated. They are looking for that second opinion and it doesn't have to be all the way down into a quaternary care process. Projects are looking at providing that second opinion without traveling the 4,000 to 8,000 miles necessary to get it in the past.

Mrs. MORELLA. Are we adequately patenting what we are doing?

Dr. TANGALOS. We are selling a service and I think we have the world leadership in medical capabilities and in services that we can provide. Commerce is very interested in the services that we are selling and I hope that we can continue to do that on a greater and greater basis. I would like to see that within the country we keep up and allow ourselves to do that as easily as we probably can internationally.

Mrs. MORELLA. You think we can work out licensing, security, confidentiality, malpractice, tort reform?

Dr. JAY SANDERS. I have addressed that in some of the handout material. The licensing to me is—we have an archaic system in the United States and I am probably going to get killed for saying this. We have all graduated taking national examinations. I would not treat a pneumonia that you might get differently in Georgia than I would in Rochester, Minnesota; yet I have to have separate licenses in Minnesota and in Georgia.

With telemedicine, there is an immediate assumption that if you are in Minnesota and I am in Georgia and I am seeing you in consultation, that I have been transmitted, I, the physician, have been transmitted to you the patient in Minnesota. Well, if that is the case and I don't have a license in Minnesota, that is a felony on my part.

However, let's flip the coin and let's say, why are you looking at it in a fashion that the doctor is being electronically transported to the patient? Why not look at it from the standpoint of the patient being transported to the doctor? Then I am practicing in Georgia where I have a license. That is one way to look at it.

A better way to look at it is to deal with the whole issue of individual state licenses and say that was a system that may have been appropriate years ago, but there is no reality to it today, and at the very least, for those people who are doing telemedicine consultations to the underserved where there is a need to provide them some sort of leeway or some sort of national licensure for telemedicine for the underserved population that are being served.

Dr. TANGALOS. We already have exclusivity built into a number of state guidelines that have considered telemedicine and say we don't want our x-rays read by out-of-state physicians. We build that into the structure of state rules and licenses.

What Dr. Koop was talking about in terms of telemedicine delivering access is when you envision a national system, it should allow every citizen in this country to access whatever appropriate medical care they need, irrespective of hard boundaries, State lines, peculiar state licensing requirements; but even within medicine, we already have the boundaries developing for those that have telemedicine opportunities and those that don't.

The question of competition, what should be, what shouldn't be are issues that are coming to the forefront and will be on the table for the next couple of years.

Mrs. MORELLA. I want to thank you, Mr. Chairman, for allowing me so much time to ask the questions. I think the panel has been superb.

Mr. HAYES. Let me also make a comment having listened to the answers. It is clear that whether you wish to be or not, and whether we wish to be or not we get drawn into some of the communications issues on competitive systems. Whether we get into telephone lines or transmission or whether we get into the cable industry and their own war, in effect you have become a part of, willing or not.

It also means that we better be careful when we look at the resolution of those issues and any changes that are made to be certain that we have left the door open for whatever health care industry best fits whatever national policy on telecommunications will operate. You mentioned cable.

You are going to hear from a rural doctor who will tell you about a place where cable isn't conceived of the same way that most of you use it. Plus, he is in a storm system. One of the reasons it was so important to have television that was non-cable was because in this remote area, during bad weather periods much less severe storms, which are quite common, that link is gone.

As we craft a system we will have to make sure that we don't have extended periods of time to which this will back up once we begin to rely more heavily on it. Thank you again. Your appearance has been most informative.

It is probably just as appropriate that Dr. Puskin has joined this panel rather than the panel you were intended for, because with your office of rural policy at HHS, it is probably as appropriate as it would have been earlier in the day. We very much appreciate your having joined us at this time.

I don't know whether you and Dr. Sanders had an order in which you wish to proceed. It doesn't matter to the committee. I guess we will start with you and work our way down the table.

STATEMENT OF GARY M. RAVETTO, CHIEF EXECUTIVE OFFICER, SOUTHWEST LOUISIANA AREA HEALTH EDUCATION CENTER, LAFAYETTE, LA

Mr. RAVETTO. That is great. Thank you. First, I too would like to thank you for this opportunity. I was looking at all the panelists and realized I am the only person here today who is not a doctor. I come from a marketing and community development background. I guess my approach to this is somewhat different than what you might have heard earlier.

I have to say that representing the agency that I do, the Area Health Education Center that serves 13 communities in southwest Louisiana, I think the idea of telemedicine and information highways is extremely important and we support it fully.

Given my background, I guess I am more of a practicalist and because of my background in marketing, I am very much customer oriented in what people need and what they perceive to be true.

As we look at national health care reform, a few realities come to mind. One is that the perception that has developed among rural communities and in particular in southwest Louisiana is that the urban health care system has grown stronger and richer while the rural system has fallen into serious crisis in large part because there are too few doctors, and those who are out there are aging and not being replaced at a proper speed.

Specifically, in southwest Louisiana, 26 percent of our primary care physicians that are currently practicing are age 65 or older. That means that not only do we have a shortage of primary physicians, but that a quarter of them who are out there are within five to ten years of retirement.

As you will hear from Dr. Sanders who can tell you from first-hand experience, they work very long hours with little or no relief. Rural hospitals compete with their larger urban counterpart facilities for patients. The perception out there is that it must be better if it is in the big city so, therefore, if I can, I will trek there and go to those facilities.

The challenges that we in my organization and my colleagues across the country face as we try to overcome this shortage is that medical schools are not encouraging rural practice in primary care. Many give lip service to doing it but the reality is that it is not happening. If it was happening, then we wouldn't need to exist and we wouldn't be talking about shortages. If we can recruit them, we have another challenge to overcome, the idea of isolation.

Telemedicine fits in well with that. It is difficult to say to a young physician just getting out of medical school or one that wants to relocate from an urban or a semi-urban area to a rural community that we can provide you with a backup if he or she is one of two physicians in the community, also the idea of long hours and lower pay and less money.

Small towns in America are very much like our cities, that is that they are individuals. I grew up in suburban Pittsburgh and spent almost a decade in Memphis, Tennessee and another four years in Houston Texas. Each community is very different, they have their own flavor and quality of life, while they are very much the same.

We hear about crime and homelessness, et cetera, but I don't hear much talk about rural America being individual. We sort of clump it. We say rural America, but I can tell you that Kaplan, Louisiana, where I have spent a lot of time, is very much the same but also very different from Kittanning, Pennsylvania, an area that I am very familiar with. We tend to forget that.

I was glad to hear testimony that telemedicine's system is such that it can be adapted to each community and to each specific need. I think that is very important. I think that anything we look at has to take into account that each community is very different culturally, economically, and they have goals and hopes for their future, what they would like to see or become or they want to be and it has to come into play.

We also know that rural America is an aging population. They tend to be older and poorer. They also tend to have a sense to feel more comfortable sticking closer to home. Those of us who live in urban communities don't feel it is unusual for us to get in our car and get on the Beltway to drive what is perceived to be across town but really is on the other side of nowhere to obtain services if we need to do that. But it is a major problem for someone particularly elderly on a fixed income to drive 25 miles to the nearest larger hospital.

How can telemedicine help? I mentioned access to care beyond the community. It will bring home to folks care and services that they cannot access right now and keep them there. And as I also mentioned, it will eliminate I hope or help to eliminate isolation and will help us in the recruitment and retention of primary care physicians, that we can keep them there because they will have a network.

I think it will help bring more revenue into these rural hospitals. They are struggling to stay alive on a day-to-day basis. If you have ever attended a rural hospital board meeting, and I have attended many, they are half a step away from closing their doors. When I first took the job, in Louisiana, we have parishes and the rest of the country has counties.

I went to the local governments to their meetings and most of the hospitals in rural America are owned by the local municipality. I made my presentation about our agency and I asked them a question—I am curious—tell me what the economic impact is of your hospital. There was not one community out of the 11 strictly rural communities that I went to, two of which, Lake Charles and Lafayette we consider urban—I don't think by financial standards, they are—but that could tell me what the economic impact was of the facility.

I was amazed because, in many communities, if it isn't the largest employer, it certainly has a large payroll that affects that communities. Rural communities, many of which are just now realizing the importance of that health care system within their community, are trying to do something about it. In many cases, it is a lot too late.

What we face—and, again, I have to share some realities—up here in Washington when we deregulated and made some changes to the cable industry and we talked about the wireless cable system, my phone rang off the wall for probably four or five months from new start-up for-profit entities to nonprofit agencies that were jumping on the bandwagon and everybody wanted to get involved.

I got phone calls from the two universities and the one satellite campus and several vocational technology schools in my area who were being wooed to get involved in these endeavors. Their heads were spinning. I see the same thing happening in the telemedicine area.

In the bureaucratic arena, we have the Governor's Office of Rural Development who is involved in spearheading an effort. We have the Department of Health and Hospitals who is involved in it. We have the charity hospitals managed by the Health Care Authority that is now involved. Not only are state universities, but the medical schools that have two campuses, one in the southern part of the State and one in the northern part of the State.

And I learned two weeks ago that they are not working together on an effort. They are working competitively on an effort. I was amazed because I attended several functions in my area of the

State where the medical schools, both of them, in a week's time wooed the same hospitals to tie into their telemedicine networks. They are just overwhelmed by this.

You have a rural health care system that is already understaffed, overworked and very, very short on money that is being wooed in all different directions. The perception is there is a reason why these guys are interested in me and I don't believe it is because they really care about me. They are interested in me like they have been in the past because there is a way for them to make more money or to get more money. That may or may not be true. That is their perception, so they are very leery about getting involved and not sure which is the best way to go.

I was pleased to hear the discussion earlier about breaking down barriers so rural providers or rural facilities could work outside of their State lines. Dr. Sanders' community is very close to the Texas border and there is a link to Galveston and to the far reaches of east Texas. It is more natural for these folks, then, to look to that part of the country for that care. If he can't do that, I think it would be a deterrent.

The same thing is true in north Louisiana. I was in Bernice, 20 miles from the Arkansas border. Board members in that hospital, which is half a step away from closing and probably will by the end of the year, told me that their market is Arkansas that they are losing to. So that if linkages could be made there, it makes sense.

However, the reality of the political climate in Louisiana, and I don't think it is unique in Louisiana—colleagues elsewhere tell me that what they see is that with health care reform and all the interest in Washington, there is going to be a lot of Federal money available so we are going to jump on that bandwagon as fast as we can and make sure that we can control or manage this kind of system.

I talked about the bureaucracies in the State that are very interested in telemedicine. I won't begin to tell you about the for-profits that have contacted my office or contacted the facilities that I serve and the providers that I serve. Everybody is very interested in it.

In light of all that, about three years ago, we have said to the powers that be in the state that we felt that it was very necessary that there be some kind of needs assessment done. Some of my staff went to Georgia and looked at the final work being done there and we have talked to several other States. Everyone told us, start with a study, find out what the providers need, what they want, what their level of knowledge and acceptance is so you know where to begin.

Area health education centers in the state just completed what we hope to be a comprehensive needs assessment. That should be ready by the middle of the month. We did four different surveys. We surveyed rural facilities, urban facilities, rural providers and urban providers.

We surveyed about 8,000 total, and one of the things that we did is to ensure its integrity. We insisted that the tool be constructed by and tabulated by a third party outside of the state so that no one could make the case such and such tabulated that data and, therefore, they have an interest in it.

81-951 O - 94 - 5

Once it was widely known that we were doing it, all the entities that I mentioned contacted us and offered to tabulate the data free of charge. We gave it to them and told them they were welcome to use the data as they saw fit, but that we were going to a third party to do that.

The majority of those surveyed agreed that telemedicine in short can help them very much and they are very eager to see a system put in place or incentives and regulations established so that they can move forward. But they are leery because of all this influx of interests coming from outside.

If telemedicine is to be an effective tool in helping to reform the American health care system, and in particular in rural areas, I believe that it must be sensitive to the needs and challenges of rural providers and facilities. The establishment of any network must be free, as free as possible of local, State and Federal politics. It needs to be unpolitical as much as possible, if it is really to do some good.

And I feel the game—what you do is pick the scapegoat, the scapegoat is always the person not in the room at the time. I feel we are doing that today, but I really feel that it needs to be as free of politics on the local and the State level. You find in States, and particularly in localities, they see a lot of money and they find ways to channel those funds into other things or to keep other things going and, therefore, its effectiveness is diluted.

In dealing with Congressman Hayes and his folks and the Senators that represent our state, I find that you come here with the very best of intentions and put things in place that you ideally and sometimes naively believe will really help those of us who live in rural communities and something happens between what you do on the Hill and what comes down to Creole, Louisiana.

In looking backwards, I have found it gets diluted as it moves in the Federal to State to local government and then to the average citizen. We have to work through that to ensure that it doesn't become diluted and distracted, that the system must always be guided by the changing demands of rural health care. It changes.

Just as it does in urban communities, rural communities change. Southwest Louisiana is having economic resurgence and is healthy right now. We hope it stays that way. It wasn't always that way, and it may change in five years. We have to adopt to that.

Finally, that the ultimate goal always be to keep strong our rural health care system and that the rural health care system is different from the urban health care system. The needs are very, very different.

To recap, if you could use these five things to guide you, that it be sensitive to rural doctors and rural hospitals, free and unpolitical, that it be managed as nonpartisanly as possible, that any changes or new regulations always be in the best interest of rural health care, and that you always ask yourself as you move along, is it truly strengthening our rural health care system.

[The prepared statement of Mr. Ravetto follows:]

This written testimony is provided by
Gary M. Ravetto-CEO/Director for
Southwest Louisiana Area
Health Education Center

Southwest Louisiana Health Education Center (SWLAHEC) is one of four area health education centers in the state. The Louisiana AHEC system identifies specific community needs, utilizing an advisory committee of health professionals, educators, and concerned citizens.

Through development of regional AHEC offices and affiliated Learning Resource Centers, LAHEC strives to improve the quality of health services available statewide. Each regional LAHEC is independently operated, allowing for customized programming to fit the needs of its service area.

SWLAHEC provides services to rural swampland communities. Except for interstate 10, the majority of the roads in this area are two-lane streets. SWLAHEC is the training and information resource for 32 hospitals and their health professionals in 13 rural parishes of the state. These parishes are: Acadia, Allen, Beauregard, Calcasieu, Cameron, Evangeline, Iberia, Jefferson Davis, Lafayette, St. Landry, St. Martin, St. Mary, and Vermilion.

SWLAHEC has formed a partnership between the educational and medical communities within these regions. The goals of the partnership are to:

* Produce and support continuing education programs for health professionals;
* Develop and implement programs which encourage health professionals to practice in rural or underserved communities of the Southwest Louisiana region;
* Establish and maintain a regional Learning Resource Center which provides Southwest Louisiana health professionals and students with current and vital medical information;
* Create and administer programs which encourage high school students, especially minorities and special-needs students, to enter health professions;
* Coordinate training programs for students of medicine, dentistry, nursing, and allied health professions.

Two years ago SWLAHEC was asked by the State of Louisiana to help in promoting the idea of a telecommunications project. The administration of SWLAHEC agreed to help because we know how telecommunications can aid in the survival of rural hospitals and practioners. Since that time, SWLAHEC has been actively involved getting acceptance of the idea of telecommunications by meeting with area health care providers and health care facilitators.

Four Louisiana Area Health Education Centers came together in a joint effort concerning a statewide survey on the possibilities of a telemedicine network in Louisiana. Telemedicine consists of basic types of interlink communication between larger urban hospitals and small rural facilities. This technology would aid in the diagnosis and treatment of patients in rural communities, both in everyday practice and emergencies, without the travel time or expense of transporting them to a larger medical complex. A telemedicine network could play a meaningful role in the plans that provide universal access of health care to rural areas in Louisiana.

Four different surveys were recently released with complete results expected by the middle of May. Surveys were mailed to specific segments of the health care industry. An estimated 8,000 individuals will be surveyed including rural and urban hospital administrators and both practicing rural and urban doctors.

The results of the study are projected to provide competent background information for the creation and implementation of a telemedicine system. The results will also be presented to the governor and his task force on telemedicine. The AHEC's effort with this survey is the only such undertaking in the state and is the only comprehensive study to be conducted in the nation.

The survey tool used in this endeavor was developed by Hezel Associates, a firm working out of New York. The survey took two and a half months to create from lack of previous research since no other state has done such an in-depth study.

Preliminary Results from LAHEC Telemedicine Needs Assessment Survey

* The majority of both the health care providers and health facility administrators were familiar with the applications of telecommunications.

  * While the majority of both groups were not currently exploring the use of telecommunications, they agreed the need for the development of advances in telecommunications initiatives is extremely important for the improvement of health delivery services in Louisiana.

  * The benefits of improved quality of service and cost savings are the reasons why some health facility administrators were exploring the use of advanced telecommunications.

  * More than half of those surveyed received their ongoing health/medical education in the form of books, journals, and non-credit workshops.

  * The principle reasons most had not enrolled in some courses they needed to take was because cost is too high and they do not have enough time.

  * Most agreed they would prefer taking workshops and courses with other health or medical professionals.

  * They also felt it was very important for them to be able to ask questions or make comments while the workshop was in progress.

  * The majority preferred, if they had the option, to take workshops and courses at a health or medical center in their community.

Data on Telecommunications

Importance of Telecommunications

* Telecommunications is vital to the recruitment and retention of health care professionals in rural areas to diminish the isolation of these areas.

* Telecommunications provide an incentive for doctors to maintain their practices in rural areas.

* Telecommunications allows for health care providers to efficiently keep up with a rapidly changing body of knowledge.

* Telecommunications helps to break down the barriers of distance to doctors in rural areas by giving them the opportunity to speak with other providers directly and to ask questions to those who may be more knowledgeable in a particular area.

* Most patients who have been involved in a telecommunications procedure have been pleased with the results.

* Telecommunications allow doctors to get immediate feedback in some cases that are life or death oriented.

Management of Telecommunications Network

* The network should take into consideration the special needs and situations hospitals work in.

* The network should allow the rural hospitals to operate with the tertiary-care centers of their choice.

* Any reimbursements should take into account the unique environment the hospital operates in.

* Any systems management of networks within states and regions should be managed by non-partisan, non-political agencies. These systems should be managed by someone who cares about the business.

Benefits of Telecommunications

* When patients are treated in their own community rather than transferred to a regional hospital, their physicians are able to provide continuity of care. This also helps to cut down on the cost of transportation for repeated trips to urban areas for follow-up care.

* Through telecommunications the latest advances in diagnoses and treatment are made available to urban health care professionals as well as rural health care professionals.

* As rural area facilities become better equipped to care for their patients, more physicians and health care dollars will remain in these smaller, isolated areas.

* Telecommunications provides immediate access to medical expertise no matter where the patient is located.

Mr. HAYES. Thank you. I was thinking that our Dr. Sanders from Creole and Dr. Sanders from Augusta could not have a more different perspective of the word medicine and practitioner.

Before Dr. Sanders begins, the area in which Dr. Sanders lives has always had the need to recruit almost any kind of expertise. From the 1930s on, it was an oil rich area. It is the coastal line of Louisiana. It is the largest parish in the State of Louisiana and has the smallest population.

For that reason, it was always difficult to recruit teachers because there weren't communities from which to recruit, and they didn't have a large enough population going to other institutions of higher learning to return home. There weren't enough folks at home to come back there. So it was very common for school boards or governmental entities to try to bring people with expertise in.

Dr. Sanders is exactly that example. He is brought in as the only physician in an area that, by itself, produces 24 percent of the seafood consumed in the United States and has a larger commercial fishing fleet than Japan and yet, at the same time, it has unquestionably as bad a north-south and east-west road link as you can imagine.

When Hurricane Audrey in 1957 hit the coastline of Louisiana, it was destructive because communications weren't as good, but the roadways, the physical system of evacuating were so bad that many people were lost in that storm simply because there wasn't a way out. It would be much better today, but if a storm that size were to hit again, it is still true, we would have casualties there solely because of lack of infrastructure.

If you understand where he comes from, you will understand even better how I wanted him here, not because he is from my home congressional district, but because he is the best example I can think of the rural physician end of this.

Mrs. MORELLA. Congressman Hayes has teased me because Maryland is for Crabs, but we have many of our crab places that are importing crabs from Louisiana. Welcome.

STATEMENT OF DR. RICHARD DUNN SANDERS, M.D., CREOLE, LA

Dr. RICHARD SANDERS. I will give a thumbnail sketch of myself. I am a rural physician. I am Richard Sanders, born in Memphis, Tennessee. I grew up in northeast Arkansas in a town called Lepanto where my father was a dentist there. I graduated from the University of Arkansas in 1975, School of Medicine. Dr. Elders was an instructor of mine there at the time. I then moved to Louisiana.

I finished a family practice residency at Moss Regional Hospital in Lake Charles in 1978. Following this, I entered the Air Force, where I served out a commitment and was honorably discharged in 1980. On October 28, 1980, when I was discharged, I set up a solo practice in Creole, Louisiana where I now am. I was recruited by the state representative there, Representative Conway LeBleu.

I have become recertified in family practice in 1985 and in also 1992 and am currently certified in family practice, board certified.

Just kind of a thumbnail sketch of the parish where I am located. We are rural, in southwest Louisiana. We are 45 miles to the next city of anything and that is Lake Charles. We are 48 miles to the next health care facility including drug store, doctor's office, hospital, anything.

The hospital which I currently am associated with South Cameron Memorial Hospital, is owned by our parish. It is a 30-bed facility with an acute care section. We also have a full-time emergency room as we have to have in that area, and we are currently operating a chemical dependency unit where we are treating cocaine addicts along with alcohol and other substance abusers.

Currently, we are adding a small nursing home on to our hospital to take care of some of our elderly. Currently, I am the only active practicing physician in our parish. In February, our other actively practicing physician died of a heart attack.

There are about 9,700 people who live in our parish. We have a large transient population which come through with fishing fleets and the oil fields and from the shrimp industry back and forth. We are located right on the Gulf of Mexico at the corner of where Louisiana and Texas run into each other.

Our economic activity is primarily oil and natural gas related, but also we have a very large commercial fleet. In addition, some of the other industries that we have there are the cattle industry, we have alligator farming, and a trapping and hunting industry there which are very big.

I mention this to show you this is somewhat unique. You don't, as Dr. Gomez and I talked about—he is from a rural area of New Mexico, but they don't have alligator farms there. The patients I see in my practice and in the emergency room range from some of the most trivial sore throat complaints, just feeling bad, to a huge variety. I have had alligator bites.

About one month ago, I had a man who was at the Rockefeller Refuge. They were trying to tag an alligator and he wasn't properly secured and he got loose, flipped over on his stomach and had the man underneath him, had the man's arm and shoulder in his mouth and was biting on it. Fortunately for the man, only a finger was lost for that.

We have schizophrenic, homeless people who have managed to wander down there. They don't know where they are and people have dumped them there. Many times the Sheriff's Department picks them up and they don't know what to do with them. They just drop them, and we have to find a mental health facility to take care of these people.

We have emergency infant deliveries. You can't very well tell a woman to hold, to wait to get to the hospital to deliver a baby when she is having it right there.

We have had to amputate a man's arm on an oil rig. We had to leave the hospital to do this. A block fell off a rig one time, pinned his arm there. The man was unconscious and he was pinned to the rig by his arm which was hanging there. We had to amputate that and get him off the rig to try to save his life.

One time I was sitting in my office talking to a patient about the weather and the back door, a woman ran in with a nine-year-old son who had quit breathing. The child had been burned approximately two weeks earlier, had been released from the hospital in another area, had respiratory distress and quit breathing. We have to do right there, do what we can to try and save that child or anybody else that comes in like this.

We have had extensive animal bites. We see quite a few injuries. Some of the illnesses that I see in the area are very unique. One illness that probably no one here except possibly Representative Hayes has heard about and duck hunters, nutraitch which is a not life threatening, but which is a larvae infection of the skin.

We see oyster illnesses from people eating oysters constantly that are out of season or spoiled or contaminated. We have a large population of migrant workers and we have a lot of immigrants from Laos, Cambodia and Vietnam in the area. This makes it unique in the way that we treat our patients. Sometimes we have cultural and communication barriers.

Talking about telecommunication, it would be good to—if I could have someone in telecommunication who could talk to these people and translate back forth.

We have many workers from Mexico, Guatemala, and Central America. I am not fluent in Spanish and usually I put the phone in their ear and call up a lady who translates for me. It would be nice to have a telecommunication network to be able to talk back and forth with each other and have it translated properly. Also to say nothing of the fact they are having to tell their illness to the community when they do this.

One of the things that I wanted to bring up was how could this save money, telemedicine. There are several things that I see that would do this. Whenever we get an old person who comes into the emergency room who has passed out, for example, you do a physical exam and one of the things you always will do is you will put your stethoscope up to their neck and hear what is known as a bruit if it exists.

A bruit is a noise in the neck and might indicate that they have obstruction in the carotid arteries. If they have a significant obstruction in the carotid arteries, immediate surgery might prevent a stroke. It would be good if we could have a probe put up to their neck and immediately transmit this image to a radiologist or to a vascular surgeon such as Dr. Gomez and have them tell me if it is dynamically significant; in other words, is that the cause of their fainting episode or is this just something that we are hearing there.

Also, every woman who has ever been pregnant has been worried when she was not feeling her baby kick. Consequently, she will call her obstetrician on the phone and he will tell her to come in, and even if you are in Bethesda, you are talking about minimum of two hours by the time he uses ultrasound and can reassure you the baby is in good shape.

It would be good in our area if you could take that probe, place it on the woman's abdomen, transmit the signal to her obstetrician and reassure the lady and yourself that there is no fetal distress, that the baby is in good shape. That would save money right there from having to transport a patient.

We frequently, as general practitioners and family practitioners, see children who come in with heart murmurs. We don't know if these heart murmurs are significant or if they are trivial or benign. Most of the time, you can tell, but sometimes you can't. It would be very good if you could talk to a pediatric cardiologist over the phone, he could tell you is this a benign murmur or does it need to be referred. If it doesn't need to be referred, you have saved a fortune for the patient right there.

In the community where I live, we have a large incidence of Marfan's syndrome. They tend to have heart trouble. It would be good if you could monitor their heart valves on a six-month or yearly basis. This would keep them from having to see cardiologist, and when you do find something significant in the deterioration of their valve, then you would know when to refer them to the cardiologist. That would save money in itself.

One other thing is whenever a patient would come to you with something such as a renal stone, you could do an IVP. Although I can read an IVP to an extent, I am not a radiologist or an expert on that. But I would like to have a urologist to tell me how long to wait on the stone to move before he has to intervene surgically.

I could keep him in my facility and keep the money there, but in addition, one thing not pointed out, the hospital I use currently has a charge of $160 a day per room. The next nearest facility charges $380 a day for a room. There is a significant savings right there if you are keeping the patient in our hospital as opposed to transferring him to another facility.

These are some of the things that telemedicine would save money on. In addition, it would help me in that I could listen to lectures that are coming out of medical schools. When I am examining the patient, the doctor who would be talking to me would be educating me while I am examining the patient. If I wanted to listen to a lecture by the head of surgery at the University of California, San Francisco, I could do so. If I wanted to listen to Mayo Clinic's internal medicine lecture or make a case presentation, I could do so. It would be good also if I had a television guide of where the different lectures were and could listen to these as I need to on education with this.

In conclusion, I want to say that even though we have heard about the virtual reality, telemedicine is not going to put a stitch in a child laceration, is not going to take a fish hook out of their face. He is not going to deal with a hallucinating psychotic and sedate him. The doctor there will have to get out of his bed in the middle of the night to take care of this, but it definitely will help.

I am a physician in a rural area, but more importantly, I consider myself a citizen of a rural area and I want what is best for my family and my community.

Thank you.

[The prepared statement of Dr. Sanders follows:]

My name is Richard Dunn Sanders. I was born in Memphis, Tenn. on July 20, 1951. I grew up in rural northeast Arkansas in the town of Lepanto where my father was a dentist. I graduated from the University of Arkansas Medical School in Little Rock in 1975. I completed a family pratice residency at Moss Regional Hosp. in Lake Charles, La.in 1978. This residency was through L.S.U. I then entered the United States Air Force and was honorably discharged with the rank of Captain in1980. I was recruited by Rep. Conway LeBleu, state representative for Cameron Parish, to set up a solo practice in Creole, Cameron Parish, La. I was board certified in Family Practice in 1978 and recertified in 1985 and 1992,

Cameron Parish is a rural parish located in southwest La. We are 45 miles from the city of Lake Charles. The hospital, South Cameron Memorial, is a 30 bed facility with a full time emergency room and Chemical Dependency unit along with acute care. We are currently building a nursing home facility as well.

I am currently the ONLY actively practicing physician in Cameron Parish. The population is approximately 9700.

My hospital is located on the Gulf of Mexico and is 48 miles from any other medical facility.

The economic activity in Cameron Parish is primarily oil industry related. There is also a large commercial fishing fleet on a seasonal basis. Some other area industries are: cattle, alligator farming, trapping and hunting.

The patients I see in my pratice and in the emergency room range from the most trivial sore throat complaints to life threatening illness, such as myocardial infarctions and auto accidents. I have seen variety of cases, including alligator bites, drug addicts,extensive burns, emergency infant delivery, schizophrenic homeless and accidents requiring immediate surgery. I have had to amputate a man's arm on the floor of a drilling rig in order to extricate him from the crown block which fell on him.

My hospital treats all patients, regardless of ability to pay. I treat pediatric, geriatric, and adults with acute illnesses. I also treat cocaine addicts and alcoholics. Due to the remoteness of my hospital I must treat every patient that comes in because there is no other doctor.

I am the only physician on the staff. I do not have any back-up. Telemedicine would help me tremendoussly by allowing me to seek consultation. I could transmit X-rays and cardiac monitor strips to a specialist and seek advice. I could use a telemedicine system to enhance my medical education by listening in on lectures at medical schools and teaching hospitals.

Telemedicine will not put a stitch in a laceration, pull a fish hook out of a child's face or sedate a hallucinating psychotic but it will help me to deal with complicated cases. I am married and have two children. I want the best for my own family as well as my community.

Mr. HAYES. Thanks very much.

You probably have heard a little bit differently as to daily occurrences than the usual panel in which you participate. Thanks for coming. Thanks for joining us, and we would very much like to conclude today's testimony, though we will have some questions, with your remarks from your earlier panel. But like I say, I think it is more interesting to have you on this one than had you been on the earlier panel. Thanks for coming.

STATEMENT OF DR. DENA S. PUSKIN, SC.D., DEPUTY DIRECTOR, OFFICE OF RURAL HEALTH POLICY, DEPARTMENT OF HEALTH AND HUMAN SERVICES, WASHINGTON, DC

Dr. PUSKIN. It is my pleasure. I am Dena Puskin, Deputy Director of the Office of Rural Health Policy, which you have heard alluded to previously. The office was created in 1987 to provide a focal point within the Department of Health and Human Services for rural health policy issues. As such, we work both with the private sector and all segments of government at the State, local and Federal levels to promote solutions to overcoming barriers to health care in rural communities.

Over the past six years, I have had the pleasure of working with rural communities to develop telemedicine projects and have seen firsthand the potential of this technology.

I wish to congratulate you for organizing this hearing. Hearings like this help us all to understand how we can translate this potential into reality.

I have been asked to provide a brief overview of telemedicine and how it might help improve health care in rural communities. I think you have heard from the other panels a lot of personal views on how this could happen.

My views are based on some of our experience in running these programs. What I would like to do today is share with you what we have learned: Let me first start with the reality of rural America. You have heard some of it here, and I think I have heard alluded to the diversity of rural America, in the sense that health care in rural America ranges from the isolated rural practitioners in Cuba, New Mexico, and where Dr. Sanders lives, where there may be 200 miles in which there are more roadrunners than there are people—to small towns in Upstate New York where in fact the population is fairly dense, where I come from, to Aspen, Colorado where, in fact, it is reasonably dense and there are certainly no economic needs there of any great import. All these communities can benefit from telemedicine, but their needs and ability to pay for it differ.

Moreover, it is clear that telemedicine systems cannot be developed in a vacuum. They have to be tied to the development of integrated systems of care to maximize their benefits. As one component of an integrated health care system, telemedicine can establish vital links between isolated providers and multi-specialty clinics benefiting all.

The first thing I would like to sort of say in connection with this is that telemedicine will not replace the rural practitioner. It is a useful adjunct to the services that these practitioners provide, but I agree with Dr. Sanders that, in no way, is it going to replace the need for practitioners in rural communities. I think there is a lot of fear on the part of rural communities that when people talk about telemedicine, they are talking about it as an excuse for not meeting the needs that they have out for practitioners. I think we need to be very, very careful about this.

What I would like to do today is just summarize some of the considerations that need to be taken into account when looking at successful systems: I also would like to provide a little bit of a perspective on where I think we are going.

First, we must recognize that telemedicine is not an end in itself, but a means to break down barriers to patient care and patient and professional education. It is the highway of the 21st Century by which we are moving information, not patients.

Second, in designing telemedicine systems we need to focus on the requirements for health care and the needs of rural communities, not the technology. Too often we become enamored with technology and lose sight of the needs of those communities. This will lead to sure failure.

For example, in the 1970s, where I go back that far in health care, the Federal Government provided a great deal of funding to upgrade rural hospitals. Many rural hospitals bought state-of-the-art equipment, especially radiology equipment, only to place it in closets after one or two uses. Basically they didn't have the people who knew how to use it, nor did they really have the use for that type of equipment.

In many rural areas what we need, rather than state-of-the-art equipment, is to start with 911 capability. That is, basic emergency care capability, which may or may not involve state-of-the-art equipment.

Technology advances have changed what we can do, and will continue to do so. The revolution in digital technology allows us to send images across miles of ordinary telephone lines, something we couldn't even dream of 21 years ago. Decreases in cost make things possible that 10 years ago would have only been available in Eric's shop at the Mayo Clinic or the Massachusetts General Hospital.

For example, codecs, which help transmit digital images and cost $100,000 five years ago, now cost less than $25,000, making this a much more affordable technology in terms of basic equipment.

The choices in technology, coupled with the variety of medical applications, create an overwhelming range of options for people to choose from. But often rural communities lack the expertise to make those choices. They need more technical assistance in order to help them and it must be objective, not your neighborhood vendor, shall we say.

Lack of adequate telecommunications infrastructure is a key barrier to diffusion of telemedicine in rural areas. As the basic cost of acquiring the equipment and the technology come down, transmission costs and other operating costs remain a major obstacle to communities implementing telemedicine systems.

For example, when the Mednet project, which we funded in West Texas, was begun, its designers found that people still had party lines. In many areas of this country, there are still party lines. They had to install what is called a dedicated T–1 line, a high-speed line, at a huge cost—$50,000 for three months, just to give you an example. Okay?

Transmission costs need to be lowered to make telemedicine economically feasible for small rural communities. As discussed by participants at our rural telemedicine workshop last November, one way to do this would be to establish a distance in sensitive telephone rate for essential services, such as health care.

Alternatively, telephone companies could create special extended service areas for health care. Tennessee has established a special rate for distance education that could be a model for what we do in health care.

And finally, telemedicine systems must be seamless to achieve economies and ease of use. That is, they must be compatible. Based on these considerations we have developed a few simple principles that we believe are necessary for a successful system.

The first is the simple system principle, KISS. Those of you in the military know what that means; It means "keep it simple, stupid." It is a familiar principle that basically says the best and most successful systems are those that use the simplest and least expensive technology to meet the need. Examples could be fax machines, good telephone networks, or the use of computer bulletin boards. These systems don't meet every need, but they meet a lot of needs for information.

A flexible system must be developed that is readily adaptable to changing technology and can take advantage of reductions in cost. User involvement is critical from the beginning of the project if you don't want to create a white elephant. Marketing to users as well as making the system user friendly is a critical component of success.

In fact, if you don't involve the users early, you are likely to find you are not going to have enough users. Or if you get one zealot, when that zealot moves away, and they often do, you find you don't have a base for the use of the equipment.

The support of administrative and professional leadership must be sought for the project to be successful. You cannot bring these projects in from the outside. You must find leadership in the communities if you are seeking rural community support. Thorough planning and coordination is necessary for successful projects. This may not sound new, but often communities get enamored with the technology, plop it in and we don't think about all the things we need to make sure it is sustainable. They also don't consider all the different ways to get the price down, such as different ways of getting transmission costs down.

Many programs are initially developed using subsidized funding from government, foundations, or industry. Those subsidies do not last forever. As part of the planning, you must say, how will this project continue in the absence of subsidies? Is it a realistic project? Are we putting in technology that cannot be sustained?

Aside from the third-party payment issue, which I would be pleased to discuss, there are many other issues regarding sustainability.

Coordination is essential. All the relevant resources in the area must be integrated and used. Rural communities need to coordinate and gain a consortium of users. If they are going to effectively use this equipment in low-density areas, they need to get multiple uses of the equipment for the phone companies to want to put it in in the first place, and to support it in the long run.

That doesn't mean that you have to put all the equipment in the school to be used for educational and medical services. What it means, is that you get together so that when you design your system, to set up an aggregate demand so it is worth putting the lines in for that community. Some people think they can put the equipment in in one place and it is going to serve all purposes. That has not been our experience. You basically do not meet the demand that way. There are special demands for health care and special demands for K through 12 education. They are not necessarily compatible in terms of time usage.

Finally, it may be self-evident, but a key component of success is training the intended users, especially those without much technical expertise. I can't emphasize enough that planners must consider the human infrastructure. In rural communities, each location needs a person on site to operate the equipment, especially when it comes to health care. It only takes one consultation where the equipment fails for many physicians to say, forget it.

Now, where, you might ask, are we today? Some of this ground has been covered by previous speakers. Suffice it to say that we are here today because there is increased interest in telemedicine.

With few exceptions, such as my office's efforts, recent Federal initiatives fund on initial capital costs, rather than the operating costs. Only now are we beginning to look at operating costs and what it really takes to systematically evaluate these systems.

For example, in March, my office announced in the Federal Register a new $4 million grant program that will focus on developing telemedicine projects contributed to an evaluation. Basically, we are looking at the role of telemedicine in fostering integrated health systems.

What you may not have heard of, because I read the previous testimony of some people and I know that program may have been mentioned, but what you may not have heard of is that the office is also planning to award a contract this fall for the initial phase of a major study to evaluate rural telemedicine projects. We will be coordinating the study with the Health Care Financing Administration which has already contracted with the Center for Health Policy Research in Denver to conduct a literature review in telemedicine and develop a framework for assessing its effectiveness.

As noted by Dr. Smits in her testimony, HCFA also has in its budget this year up to $5 million for rural telemedicine projects to examine how to pay for them. I think it is very important to say that all these projects are beginning to look at how to systematically evaluate what we are doing in telemedicine.

Now, payment for telemedicine is a hot topic. Clearly if telemedicine is to be viable in the long run, it will need to receive payment from third-party payers. However, the issues in terms of evaluating how to pay for it is very difficult.

In conclusion, as noted earlier, the electronic highway is to move information, not people. In rural communities, where distance is a major barrier to receiving quality health services, the electronic highway provides a major opportunity to improve access to health care. However, just as the interstate highway bypassed rural communities, contributing to their economic decline, many fear that the same could happen to these communities with telemedicine.

For telemedicine to realize its potential in these communities, we must assure an adequate rural telecommunications infrastructure. Given the cost of that infrastructure, however, it may be a while before it reaches our most remote rural communities. As such, we need to encourage these communities to build on their current telecommunications systems and develop cost-effective telemedicine applications starting with what they have. And there are many things that can be done.

It is our experience that the very act of developing these telemedicine systems, no matter what the current infrastructure, serves as catalyst for communities to collaborate across a wide spectrum of applications and build the market demand necessary to support more advanced telemedicine applications.

While we believe strongly in the promise of this technology for rural communities, we currently lack information that is systematically collected over a large enough sample to properly evaluate it. Without such information, we run the risk of investing Federal dollars in programs that are of limited benefit to our most needy communities.

We are committed to work with others, both in the Federal Government and outside, to develop programs that systematically collect and evaluate the information necessary to insure that these limited dollars are well spent.

I am pleased to answer any questions.

Thank you.

[The prepared statement of Dr. Puskin follows:]

Testimony of

Dena S. Puskin, Sc.D.
Deputy Director, Office of Rural Health Policy
Health Resources and Services Administration
Department of Health and Human Services
on
Rural Telemedicine

to the

Investigations and Oversight Subcommittee
House Committee on Science, Space and Technology

May 2, 1994

Mr. Chairman and Members of the Committee:

It is a pleasure to be here today. My name is Dena Puskin and I am Deputy Director of the Office of Rural Health Policy in the Health Resources and Services Administration of the Department of Health and Human Services. The Office was created in 1987 to provide a focal point within the Department for rural health policy development. The Office works both with government at federal, state, and local levels, and with the private sector to promote solutions to overcoming the barriers to quality health care in rural communities.

Over the past six years, I have had the pleasure of working with rural communities to develop telemedicine projects and have seen, first-hand, the vast potential telecommunications technology offers for improving the health care services available to rural Americans. I wish to congratulate the Committee for organizing this hearing. Hearings like this help all of us understand how we can best translate this potential into reality.

I have been asked to provide a brief overview of the applications of telemedicine for improving health care in rural communities. My comments and observations stem from our office's experience in sponsoring a number of telemedicine projects.

Through June of 1992, for example, the Office managed a Department demonstration grant that launched an interactive video system based at the Texas Tech University Health Sciences Center

-- the Mednet project. Using satellite technology, the Health Sciences Center in urban Lubbock has been linked with over 40 rural hospitals throughout Texas. Nine hours of continuing education programs per week are beamed via satellite from the center to rural physicians, nurses, and other health professionals at various sites. Medical consultations are also available (using telephone line-based T1 compressed video technology) for sites in Alpine and Presidio, which serve a large and remote area of western Texas.

In 1992, the Office awarded another telemedicine grant to West Virginia University for a similar project that links the University's Health Sciences Center in Morgantown to three rural hospitals. The Center provides 24-hour medical consultations, emergency assistance, and continuing education to the remote sites. Grand rounds from both the Health Sciences Center and the remote sites are included in the programming.

The delivery of mental health services through telecommunications technology is being demonstrated in Oregon as one of our Office's Outreach grant projects. There, a consortium of community mental health centers in 13 rural counties has hooked into an already existing satellite transmission system, used for distance education, to access mental health specialists in Portland and Pendleton, Oregon, for case management needs.

Policy and regulatory issues surrounding the rural applications of telemedicine were examined recently in an invitational workshop that we sponsored last November. Top-level specialists and policy-makers from across the nation assembled to discuss the barriers and opportunities for rural telemedicine. A summary of that workshop will be published by late May. I have brought draft copies with me today.

Newly available from the Office for those of you who, like me, confuse a bit with a byte, is a primer on rural telecommunications: *Rural Telehealth: Telemedicine, Distance Education, and Informatics for Rural Health Care*. Also available in reprint is an article prepared by me for the New York Academy of Sciences on rural telemedicine. Copies of these publications will be made available to the Committee.

What Have We Learned

Well what have we learned? First, we've learned that you have to start with the reality of rural America in developing telemedicine projects. While much of what I am about to say will be familiar to some of you, for others, the reality of health care in rural America may be limited to that gleaned from "Northern Exposure" or other television shows.

Rural health care ranges from the isolated primary care practitioner in Cuba, New Mexico, serving individuals in a 200 mile area where there are more road-runners than there are people; to the community health center in Eutaw, Alabama, whose rural population is isolated more by poverty than by distance; to the multi-specialty clinic in Aspen, Colorado, serving well-heeled clients from all over the nation and the world.

All these communities could benefit from telemedicine, but all don't have the same needs or ability to pay for it. Moreover, what has been clear to us is that telemedicine systems cannot be developed in a vacuum. They must be tied to the development of integrated systems of care if they are to achieve the promise of reducing rural physician and patient isolation. Moreover, telemedicine will never replace the rural primary care practitioner. But it can be a critical adjunct to the provision of quality health services in rural communities.

As one component of an integrated health care system, telemedicine can establish vital links between isolated rural providers and multi-specialty health care centers, accruing benefits to all participants. Patients in rural areas are afforded access to specialist services without excessive travel times and distances. Rural practitioners are able to interact with one another and with other health care providers, thereby reducing professional isolation and providing opportunities for continuing education. Rural hospitals benefit from telemedicine by being able to treat and receive payment for patients who might otherwise go to other facilities. Multi-specialty hospitals have opportunities to develop referral channels for treatment and follow-up. Moreover, telemedicine facilitates the return of rural patients to their communities at an appropriate level of care once specialty services are no longer needed.

Today, I'm going to review some major considerations in developing effective rural telemedicine systems and highlight the elements of successful systems; then summarize where we are today; and finally provide some perspective on where we might be going.
As we have gained experience with telemedicine, certain reoccurring considerations emerge.

First, we must recognize that telemedicine is not an end in itself, but a means to break down barriers to patient care and professional education. Telecommunications is the highway of the 21st century by which we are moving information, not patients.

Second, in designing telemedicine systems, we need to focus on the requirements of health care and the needs of rural communities, not the technology. Too often we become enamored with technology. This will lead to failure and disappointment in rural areas. For example, in the 1970s, the Federal government provided a great deal of funding to upgrade rural hospitals. Many rural hospitals bought "state-of-the art" radiology equipment, only to place it in closets because they did not have the staff to maintain or operate it effectively. In some rural areas, simple telecommunications services, such as "911" capability, are more significant than sophisticated equipment that sits unused most of the time.

Third, technology advances have changed what we can do ... and will continue to do so. The revolution in digital technology allows us to send images across ordinary telephone lines--something we could only dream of 20 years ago. Decreasing costs make things possible in rural areas that 10 years ago would have only been available at the Mayo Clinic or Mass General Hospital. For example, codecs that cost $100,000 just 5 years ago, now cost less than $25,000.

The choices in technology, coupled with the variety of medical applications, creates an overwhelming array of options when developing telemedicine systems. Decisions must be made with care to assure that scarce resources are spent appropriately. Often rural communities do not have adequate information and the in-house expertise to make these choices. Objective sources of technical assistance are greatly needed.

Fourth, lack of an adequate telecommunications infrastructure is a key barrier to the diffusion of telemedicine in rural areas. As the basic costs for acquiring telemedicine technology have come down, transmission costs and other operating costs remain a major obstacle to communities implementing telemedicine systems. For example, when the Mednet project began, its designers found that people still had party lines in West Texas. They had to install dedicated T1 lines at a huge cost in order to provide telemedicine services.

Transmission costs need to be lowered to make telemedicine economically feasible for small rural communities. As discussed by participants at our rural telemedicine workshop last November, one way to do this would be to establish a distance insensitive telephone rate for essential services, such as health care. Alternately, telephone companies could create special extended service areas for health care. Tennessee has established a special rate for distance education that could be a model.

And finally, telemedicine systems must be seamless to achieve economies and ease of use; that is, they must be compatible with each other to ensure they are interconnectable and flexible.

Based on these considerations, we have developed a few simple principles that we believe are key to successful telemedicine systems in rural communities.

Principles

KISS --KEEP IT SIMPLE STUPID -- a military principle familiar to many of you. Experience has led us to conclude that the most successful systems are those that use the simplest and least expensive technology to meet a need. Examples of such successful systems include use of a telephone consultation network in Alabama --Access-- or the use of computer electronic bulletin boards in Texas for computer conferencing and education programs for tumor registrars.

A **FLEXIBLE SYSTEM** must be developed that is readily adaptable to rapid changes in technology and that can take advantage of reductions in cost.

To be successful, programs must incorporate **USER INVOLVEMENT** from the beginning of the project to avoid developing a white elephant that is never used. Marketing to users, as well as making the system user friendly, is a critical component of success.

Technology is not enough; the system must be viewed as useful and must receive user support. User input is also critical to determine the levels of technology that are acceptable. For example, the quality of picture resolution that is acceptable will vary depending on whether the system is to be used for education or medical diagnosis.

The support of **ADMINISTRATIVE AND PROFESSIONAL LEADERSHIP** must be sought for the project to be successful. Projects need champions to be successful.

Thorough **PLANNING AND COORDINATION** is necessary for successful projects. The message is plan, plan, plan, and coordinate at all levels from the beginning of the project. Projects should begin with a careful analysis of the present telecommunications infrastructure and build upon it. Planners must consider modes of transmission such as microwave, copper, fiber, and satellites. They must also consider the capital and transmission costs associated with developing systems that use various modes.

Many programs are initially developed using subsidized funding from government, foundations, or industry. Continuity of service in the absence of subsidy must be planned for from a project's beginning, including careful assessment of sources for ongoing payment for operating costs. Relevant reimbursement and funding sources should be assessed early in the project's life.

Coordination is essential. All the relevant resources available in an area should be integrated and used if possible. Once again, we learned some valuable lessons from the early stages of the Mednet project. The nursing school had a program in distance education, funded by a foundation prior to the beginning of Mednet; yet this program was not integrated into the

Mednet project. As a result, Mednet spent far more for its nursing education program than was necessary.

A **CONSORTIUM** of users should be developed to promote effective use and reduce cost of infrastructure development through aggregating demand for technology. Rural communities are often too small to support the ongoing operating costs that are necessary for more sophisticated applications of telemedicine. Rural telemedicine must be viewed as part and parcel of rural development. The potential for telemedicine is greatly enhanced by aggregating demand -- that is, by communities creating systems that can be used for a variety of social service purposes -- from education to health.

And finally, although it may be self-evident, a key component of any successful telecommunications project is the training of its intended users, especially those without much technical experience. Provision for ongoing technical assistance and support is essential to the success of projects. I can't emphasize enough that planners must consider the **HUMAN INFRASTRUCTURE**. In rural communities, an indigenous person needs to be available who can operate the equipment at each rural site, so the equipment does not end up in the closet. It only takes one consultation where the equipment fails for many physicians to say, "forget it."

<u>Where are We</u>

Now where -- you well might ask -- are we today. Some of this ground has been covered by previous speakers. Suffice it to say, there is increased interest in telemedicine at the national and state levels as the nation begins to seriously address its information needs.

With few exceptions, such as my office's programs, recent Federal initiatives have tended to fund initial capital start-up costs, rather than operating costs. Only now are we seeing initiatives aimed at supporting operating costs associated with planning and implementation of these systems. Moreover, given increased interest in telemedicine, there is an increasing call to formally and systematically evaluate these systems.

For example, in March, my office announced in the Federal Register a new 4 million dollar grant program that will focus on developing telemedicine projects that will contribute to an evaluation. A central goal of the program is to demonstrate how telemedicine can be used as an effective tool in promoting integrated systems of health care in rural communities. Integral to the program is the development of an information base that will allow evaluation of the demonstration projects. The deadline for applications is May 20. My office is also planning to award a contract this fall for the initial design phase of a major study to evaluate rural telemedicine projects. We will be coordinating this study with the Health Care Financing Administration (HCFA), which has contracted with the Center for Health Policy Research (CHPR) in Denver to conduct a literature review of telemedicine and develop a framework for assessing its effectiveness.

As noted by Dr. Smits in her testimony, HCFA also has in its budget up to $5 million this year for rural telemedicine projects to begin to examine how to pay for telemedicine under federal payment programs. Payment for telemedicine is a hot topic. Clearly, if telemedicine is to be viable in the long run, it will need to receive payment from third party payers.

Conclusion

As noted earlier, the goal of the electronic highway is to move information, not people. For rural communities, where distance is a major barrier to receiving quality health services, the electronic highway provides an opportunity to improve access to health care for rural residents. However, just as the interstate highway bypassed rural communities, contributing to their economic decline, many fear that, with telemedicine, the same could happen to these communities if we are not careful. For telemedicine to realize its potential in these communities, we must assure an adequate rural telecommunications infrastructure. We must also recognize that given the cost of developing that infrastructure, it may be a while before it reaches our most remote rural communities. As such, we need to encourage these communities to build on their current telecommunications base to develop cost-effective telemedicine applications. It has been our experience that the very act of developing these telemedicine systems provides a catalyst for communities to collaborate across a wide spectrum of applications and build the market demand necessary to support more advanced telemedicine services .

While we believe strongly in the promise of this technology for rural communities, we currently lack information that is systematically collected over a large enough sample to properly evaluate it. Without such information, we run the risk of increasingly investing Federal dollars in programs that are of limited benefit to our most needy communities. We are committed to work with others, both in and out of the Federal government, to develop programs that systematically collect and evaluate the information necessary to ensure that limited Federal dollars are well spent.

I would be pleased to answer any questions you may have.

Reprinted from Extended Clinical Consulting By Hospital Computer Networks
volume 670 of the *Annals of the New York Academy of Sciences*
December 17, 1992

Telecommunications in Rural America

Opportunities and Challenges for the Health Care System

DENA S. PUSKIN

Office of Rural Health Policy
Health Resources and Services Administration
U.S. Department of Health and Human Services
Rockville, Maryland 20857

I am really pleased to be here today. My pleasure is double: first, to have a chance to spend time with so many experts on telecommunications, and second, to be able to participate in a New York Academy of Sciences conference. I have long admired the work of the Academy in promoting the spirit of free scientific inquiry through its outstanding conferences.

First, a word about the federal Office of Rural Health Policy. The Office was created in 1987 to work within the Department of Health and Human Services and with federal, state, and other entities outside of the Department to seek solutions to problems in rural communities. Among its responsibilities, the Office advises the Secretary of Health and Human Services on the effects of Medicare and Medicaid regulations on access to health care by rural residents.

Of particular interest to today's discussion is the role of the Office in sponsoring telecommunications demonstrations. Currently, the Office funds a major demonstration in West Texas, the MEDNET project. The MEDNET project is a $1.8 million effort to demonstrate the potential for reducing the isolation of rural health practitioners through the use of telecommunications for continuing education and telemedicine. In addition, we are planning to fund a telemedicine project in West Virginia that will focus more directly on assessing the cost-effectiveness and clinical acceptability of telecommunications for the diagnosis and treatment of patients in rural settings. Some of my comments today derive from our experience with these projects. In our discussion today, I will focus on the application of telecommunications technology in rural America to distance learning for health professionals and to the practice of medicine.

MAJOR THEMES

Throughout this discussion, several themes will reoccur. Although some of the themes are unique to rural communities, some are equally applicable to urban areas.

Telecommunications is not an end in itself, but a means to an end which is to break down barriers to care. The use of telecommunications in rural health care improves access to care and breaks down the barriers of distance. Telecommunication is the highway of the twenty-first century that will transmit information, not people.

Technology advances have changed what we can do. Twenty years ago, the technology basically existed only to send costly analog signals, often with poor resolution. Today, the cost-reducing technology exists to compress an analog image into digital signal, send it across telephone lines, and make the image analog again for viewing at the receiving site. The different types of telephone lines for sending information range from normal telephone lines which transmit information at 64 thousand bits/sec, to T1 and T3 lines which send transmissions at 1.5 million bits/sec and at 45 million bits/sec, respectively. Technologists speculate that they will be able to transmit a clinically acceptable image with one-quarter of a T1 line in the near future.

Furthermore, the cost of the technology is decreasing rapidly. CODEC units that just a few years ago were over $100,000 are now under $30,000. The decreasing costs have made the technology increasingly accessible to rural hospitals, whereas formerly it was only available at large medical centers such as the Mayo Clinic and Massachusetts General Hospital.

Though the majority of those looking into the use of this equipment will not admit it, they desire an image that has as high a resolution as their television sets. This is not possible with the current technology, but may soon be available.

Cost-effectiveness equation varies. A cost-effectiveness equation exists in rural telecommunications that is very different depending upon the level of infrastructure development and the expectations of the users. For example, the ability of the Mayo Clinic in Minnesota to absorb the costs incurred for a transmission to its branch clinic in Florida is significantly different than that of a small hospital in Alpine, Texas to transmit to the Texas Tech Health Sciences Center in Lubbock, Texas.

No major assessments have been made of cost-effectiveness in rural areas for medical applications. Much remains to be learned. For example, what is the level of technology (e.g., resolution) that doctors find clinically acceptable for specific types of consultations, and what does it cost to do a consult, as the costs vary with the equipment used and the costs of transmission?

Lack of adequate technology infrastructure development is a key barrier to the diffusion of telecommunications in rural communities. Infrastructure is the key to the development of telecommunications in rural areas. We need to support a telecommunications infrastructure that will sustain statewide and community-specific development goals, while keeping the services affordable and within the reach of all consumers. It also must be remembered that policy for telecommunications is established on the state and federal levels, whereas rural development activity tends to be based locally.

Human capital is the key in applying telecommunications in rural health care settings. Technology advancement and infrastructure development are necessary, but not sufficient to encourage the diffusion of telecommunications applications in rural areas. Human capital is key, and education must be sufficient to provide a skilled work force that is capable of using the technology. Basically, at all levels we are dealing with changing social and political attitudes about technology and telecommunications. We are undergoing a social revolution through technology that is especially painful for rural areas that may not have the trained work force to adapt to these changes.

Let's look more closely at some of the issues raised.

81-951 O - 94 - 6

ECONOMIC DEVELOPMENT—A KEY COMPONENT FOR MARRYING TELECOMMUNICATIONS AND HEALTH CARE

In discussions about the interrelationships between rural economic development and health care, we are faced with the proverbial "chicken and egg." We need social services to attract and retain a rural community's economic base, but we also need a sufficient economic base to retain health care services.

Economic, education, and health indicators show rural America lagging behind its urban neighbors. Two economic factors conspire to further dim the prospects for rural telemedicine. First, today's global economy forces rural communities to compete in international markets. Second, rural communities lag behind metropolitan areas in being able to access modern telecommunications.

Roads and transportation arteries linking rural regions with urban centers were once considered vital to sustaining rural life. In the past, markets for goods and services were geographically tied to specific places. We attempted to centralize production of goods in one area and distribute them to another. Economies of scale were tied to producing goods in concentrated areas.

Today, in the modern information era, telecommunications and information are just as vital as roads. They are the modern roads of commerce. What we see are emerging markets for services that are not tied to small places. Telecommunications has enlarged and diffused the area of markets for both production and distribution of goods and services by reducing time—especially when the market is for services. An example of this is Rosenbluth Travel, which has its worldwide travel services based in North Dakota, and I am told that, as a result, North Dakota is almost totally connected by fiber optics.

What we see emerging is the demand for decentralized, customized production systems that are speedy. Distance is not the key in these markets—speed of production is.

If rural America is to survive, it must take advantage of these new patterns of commerce based on telecommunications. Yet telecommunications systems depend heavily on a well-educated, talented work force; thus developing and implementing the technology in rural areas is not enough. We must have the work force that can use it. If we don't develop and support that work force, rural areas will continue to decline as places to live and work.

HEALTH CARE TRENDS

What are the parallels and implications for rural health? Before we get too deeply into the discussion of telecommunication applications for health care, it might be useful to review some recent health care trends in rural America.

Historically, rural America has always had a difficult time providing health care to its residents. The barriers of distance contribute to professional isolation, making it difficult to recruit and retain health professionals. Lower incomes and more fragile economies make it difficult to sustain health care institutions.

For this reason, federal, state, and local governments have long played a role in subsidizing health care services in rural areas. The Hill-Burton Program, throughout the 1940s, 1950s, and early 1960s, built hospitals in rural America. The National Health Service Corps in the 1970s provided scholarships for physicians and others to serve in underserved areas of the United States.

The 1980s witnessed major changes in health care. Technological development and insurers' attempts to contain health care costs acted to shift basic acute care services, including many surgical procedures, out of the hospital, while the remaining hospital inpatient care became more complex. New types of providers such as ambulatory surgical centers were established, while old-style small general hospitals began to disappear.

In a sense, the economic environment of rural hospitals became more competitive. Competition came from new kinds of providers and from urban hospitals that could provide the level of sophisticated care that rural hospitals increasingly could not. Urban hospitals generally were larger than most rural hospitals and, given their larger size, often could purchase more advanced equipment and often utilize it at a lower cost per patient. Yet, rural hospitals have been the linchpin of the rural health care system. As they close, providers often take flight, leaving these communities with little or no care.

The health professions have also undergone changes which severely affect the recruitment and retention of personnel in rural areas. Despite efforts to increase the pool of primary care physicians in the United States, physicians continue to specialize, resulting in a greater need to work in settings that support high technology care. Personnel shortages in rural areas in the 1980s were exacerbated by the decline of the rural hospital. Currently, there are approximately half the number of physicians per capita in rural compared to urban areas. The supply of mid-level practitioners who frequently practice in rural communities, such as physician assistants and nurse practitioners, has grown but the demand outstrips the growth. Furthermore, nursing and allied health care personnel shortages are seen around the country in both urban and rural areas, but it is especially difficult to recruit this personnel to rural areas.

Professional isolation is an almost insurmountable problem. Primary care physicians want specialty backup, so even if a primary care physician can be recruited, retention is difficult. Many communities have found that they cannot recruit health care personnel but must "home grow 'em."

The decline of the rural hospital together with persistent and devastating shortages of health care personnel has increased interest in health care networks that link communities together to provide care. Many of these networks include limited service institutions linked to full-service medical centers for back-up specialty and emergency care.

One example of this approach is embodied in the recently implemented federal program, the Essential Access Community Hospital (EACH). The EACH is a full-service hospital that acts as a backup for more limited and remote small hospitals, the Rural Primary Care Hospitals (RPCHs). A RPCH is a facility with no more than six beds which may use non-physician personnel to provide limited inpatient care for up to 72 hours and 24-hour emergency service availability. The EACH serves as a referral and transfer facility where physicians from the RPCH may admit and treat patients. We believe that a critical element in the success of this program will be the effective use of telecommunications. Telecommunications has the potential to promote the more effective use of non-physician personnel at the RPCH by providing them with ready consultative backup with personnel at the EACH, and thus ensuring better care for rural patients.

TELECOMMUNICATIONS—DISTANCE LEARNING AND TELEMEDICINE

We've heard a lot of discussion about sophisticated telecommunications this morning. In rural areas, the applications of telecommunications technology for health care range from the simple use of the telephone for data transmission, to use of full-motion, two-way interactive video for medical consultation.

Today, I'd like to focus on two applications of telecommunications in rural areas—distance learning and telemedicine for health professionals. In a sense, I see them as different points on a continuum of lifetime learning for health professionals.

As I noted previously, we continue to experience extreme shortages of personnel in rural areas. The provision of degree program courses and didactic continuing education through telecommunications has been shown to be an effective tool for both training and recruitment. Rural communities find that distance learning programs have helped them upgrade the skills of existing personnel and attract new personnel. This reduces the cost of travel and increases continuing education opportunities for licensure and accreditation.

Telemedicine is far less developed than distance learning in rural areas, in large part because of both the high cost and limited acceptance of telemedicine. However, where implemented, telemedicine has been shown to be an effective tool for providing medical consultation. We also believe (although scientific evaluations remain to be conducted) that telemedicine is an effective tool for reducing isolation and thereby retaining health professionals in rural areas. Moreover, we believe that for rural areas, telemedicine may prove to be the most effective tool for continuing education, especially for physicians. Telemedicine is one-on-one teaching and learning which creates ongoing relationships between professionals. Finally, telemedicine is one of the keys to forging effective networks—distance learning and telemedicine involve a variety of technologies.

Telemedicine systems run using a variety of equipment and modes of transmission. The technology may be as simple as the telephone, such as the Medical Access and Referral System (MARS) in Morgantown, West Virginia, where a toll-free 24-hour-a-day service links rural community physicians to the West Virginia University specialists or subspecialists. The system is used for more than 1,000 phone consultations each month. Facsimile machines are used for everything from the transmission of medical records and pharmaceutical orders to EKG interpretations. Electronic bulletin boards, utilizing personal computers, keep rural providers apprised of the latest information and permit them to participate in an ongoing dialogue with specialists. Compressed still-frame video technology to send radiographs is an example of a more sophisticated application of technology for medical diagnosis which allows practitioners to instantaneously share clinical information.

ELEMENTS OF A SUCCESSFUL SYSTEM

What I'd now like to share with you is my somewhat idiosyncratic view of what makes a successful rural telecommunications system (and what does not). My comments are based on our experience in the United States and on the extensive experience of Max House in Canada. They also reflect awareness of the larger market changes and skill demands I spoke of earlier, which, I believe, are inherent in modern telecommunications.

"KISS—Keep It Simple Stupid"

Experience has led us to conclude that the most successful systems are those that use the simplest and least expensive technology necessary to meet a need. Examples of such successful systems are (1) the MARS program in West Virginia which I discussed earlier; (2) the continuing education program at Northampton-Accomack Memorial Hospital in the Tidewater area of Virginia which uses public television to transmit education programs to upgrade the skills of nursing personnel; (3) use of electronic bulletin boards in Texas for computer conferencing and education programs for tumor registrars; and (4) the use of fax machines in West Texas to transmit data about a patient from the rural hospital to the consulting physician. The message here is the old axiom "keep it simple stupid—KISS."

Flexibility is Essential

A flexible system must be developed. The system must be readily adaptable to rapid changes in technology and take advantage of reductions in cost. Advances in fiber optics and compressed video technology are making this technology increasingly affordable for rural areas.

User Involvement

To be successful, programs must involve users from the beginning of the project in order to avoid developing a white elephant that is never used. Marketing to users is key, as well as making the system user friendly. As noted earlier, technology is not enough. The system must be viewed as useful, and user support is essential. Moreover, user input is critical to determine the levels of technology that are acceptable; for example, the quality of resolution that is acceptable has been shown to markedly differ if the use is for education versus medical diagnosis. In the MEDNET project, user advisory committees were established to facilitate this input.

Administrative and Professional Leadership

The support of administrative and professional leadership must be sought for the project to be successful. When there is a champion of the project in an area, it is much more likely to be used. This lesson was graphically illustrated in the MEDNET project where the telemedicine technology was used at much greater rates in Alpine than in Fort Stockton, Texas because there was a physician in Alpine who liked the technology and was involved in the project from the beginning.

Plan, Plan, Plan, and Coordinate

Thorough planning is required. Plan carefully for coordination at all levels. All of the technology available within a given area should be utilized and integrated for the most successful project. Once again, we learned a lesson from the MEDNET project. The nursing school had a program in distance education, funded with foundation funds prior to the beginning of MEDNET; yet this program was not integrated into MEDNET. As a result, the MEDNET project initially incurred much higher costs to produce its nursing programs than would have been necessary.

Promote Consortium of Users to Achieve Economies of Scale

A consortium of users should be developed to promote to effective use and reduce the cost of infrastructure development through aggregating demand for the technology. It should include, when possible, users within and outside the health field, so that the greatest benefit to the community may be reaped. Educational programs should be included, as well as a variety of programs directed at all health professionals. Furthermore, demand should be aggregated for the creation of a rural area network similar to the network developed in North Dakota.

Continuity of Service in the Absence of Subsidies

Many programs are initially developed using subsidized funding from government, foundations, or industry. Continuity of service in the absence of subsidy should be considered from the beginning of any program development. Relevant reimbursement and funding sources should be approached early in the development of the program to determine availability of ongoing funding or to determine what types of information would be needed to garner such funding.

Overcoming Regulatory Barriers

There is frequently little need for a great deal of money in the development of many telecommunications applications, although regulatory barriers often raise costs beyond the reach of many rural communities. For example, I have been told that in West Texas, within the same local access and transport area (LATA), the telephone transmission cost is $27 per mile for a T1 line, whereas between LATAs, it is $5 per mile.

Start with What You Have

When you begin planning, consider the present telecommunications infrastructure and always start with what you have. Planners must consider modes of transmission such as microwave, copper, fiber optic, and satellites. They must also consider the tariffs that accompany them. Moreover, I can't emphasize enough that planners must consider the human infrastructure. In rural communities, an indigenous person needs to be available who can operate the equipment at each rural site, so that the technology does not end up in a closet.

Pilot Projects

Pilot projects are essential prerequisites to the successful development of full-scale health care telecommunications programs. Small projects allow you to test the technology and its acceptance before entering into major financial commitments.

Human Infrastructure Development

Although it may be self-evident, a key component of any successful telecommunications project is the training of its intended users, especially those without much technical experience.

EXAMPLES FROM OUR EXPERIENCE

Alpine, Texas may be 200 rocky, sagebrush-covered miles from any major city, but it is not isolated professionally. When a family doctor gets in trouble, he or she doesn't have to send smoke signals. He calls for help by television.

In late July of 1990, a routine telemedicine consultation between Dr. James Luecke in Alpine and Dr. Marion Myers at the Health Sciences Center in Lubbock saved a baby's life. The baby was in severe respiratory distress. Dr. Myers, a neonatal specialist, reviewed the x-ray (shown over compressed video), discussed lab tests (results were faxed), and determined treatment.

What is most important to note is that Dr. Myers was so pleased with the result of the consultation that she urged Dr. Luecke to call any time he had a problem. This was the beginning of a beautiful professional relationship and network. Dr. Luecke's smile and thumbs-up told it all—that's telemedicine—immediate, interactive, personal, and lifesaving.

Similar stories are told by Sue Kwentus from the Tidewater area of Virginia about how distance learning has helped her hospital nursing staff feel they have a future in their community. As a result, they are willing to stay and work there rather than leave for the "big cities" of Richmond and Roanoke. She utilizes public television to provide nursing education programs to her staff so that they don't have to travel long distances to get the education needed for professional growth.

These are not isolated examples. They are repeated every day, more and more in rural America. Sometimes video is used, while at other times a fax or a telephone is used. Whatever the technology, more and more we are bridging the distances in health care using modern telecommunications. We hope to continue funding innovative projects such as Texas Tech's MEDNET and Mountaineer Doctor Television in West Virginia. The irony is that just when modern telecommunications and information technologies are playing an increasingly important role in business and health, the regulatory structure that once provided rural areas equal access to them is coming apart.

WHERE WE ARE TODAY

The breakup of the Bell System and the shift toward deregulated services have undermined the system of subsidies that once supported rural areas. If rural areas are not to suffer further decline, new concepts and designs for rural telecommunications must be found.

The Office of Technology Assessment has recommended the development of rural area networks which would aggregate the demand for telecommunications.

The barriers to the proliferation of telecommunications in rural areas are many. Regulations often are promoted to ensure fair competition at a time when greater collaboration is needed. Barriers also exist in terms of the type of service available, as some rural areas still have party lines, while others do have private lines but the quality is poor. The people infrastructure must not be forgotten because poor education and experience often preclude the use of the technology.

We need to bring together the major players in this area to develop a strategy of rural development. This was in part recognized by Congress in the Food, Agriculture, Conservation, and Trade Act of 1990 (Farm Bill)—P.L. 101-624, which authorized a demonstration to link development and health; to make affordable, advanced telecommunications available to rural residents, including services such as fax and data transmission, multiframing tone and signal services as well as imaging, interactive audio and video through the Rural Electrification Administration (REA).

Previously, we have had loans to upgrade phone systems through REA for telecommunications and through the Farmer's Home Administration. Limited grants have also been available. For the first time, a federal program is available which explicitly links telemedicine to rural development. This year, $5,000,000 is available in grants for medical links (planning and equipment) and distance education through the REA .

Hopefully, these demonstrations will illustrate how various technologies may be linked to achieve medical and economic synergy. By linking informatics, video, consulting, and conferencing, the opportunities are boundless.

The National Library of Medicine (NLM) is also promoting linkages through its Rural Outreach Program. Currently, NLM's National Network of Libraries of Medicine consists of eight regional medical libraries, 135 resource libraries, and 3600 member institutions. Since 1989, NLM has funded over 139 institutions and groups to introduce "Grateful Med" to rural health professionals. Grateful Med is NLM's computer software system that links health professionals to NLM's vast databases. So no matter where you live, from the remote regions of Alaska to New York City, health professionals can have access to the vast storehouse of knowledge at NLM.

In all of these efforts, an overwhelming need exists for systematic evaluation. An extensive evaluation of distance learning is needed to determine its long-term effectiveness. Further, a scientific evaluation of telemedicine is required, because previous evaluations have been self-serving, have given little information on actual costs, and do not provide adequate information on the efficacy of these technologies, especially in telemedicine. A more thorough study of what physicians find acceptable in the field and the true cost of the consultations is needed.

VISION FOR THE FUTURE

It is much easier to explain the past than predict the future. What I can say is we need a vision for telecommunications that recognizes new market forces and looks to promoting cooperative telecommunications arrangements that, in turn, foster rural development.

The states and the federal government must play a critical role in creating those incentives, but we look to you, the experts to help us d[illegible] In the end, the challenge for making modern telecommunications useful for rural America is ours and is limited only by our imagination and dedication.

Rural Health Travels the Telecommunications Highway

REACHING RURAL

A report from the Office of Rural Health Policy, Health Resources and Services Administration, Public Health Service, Department of Health and Human Services.

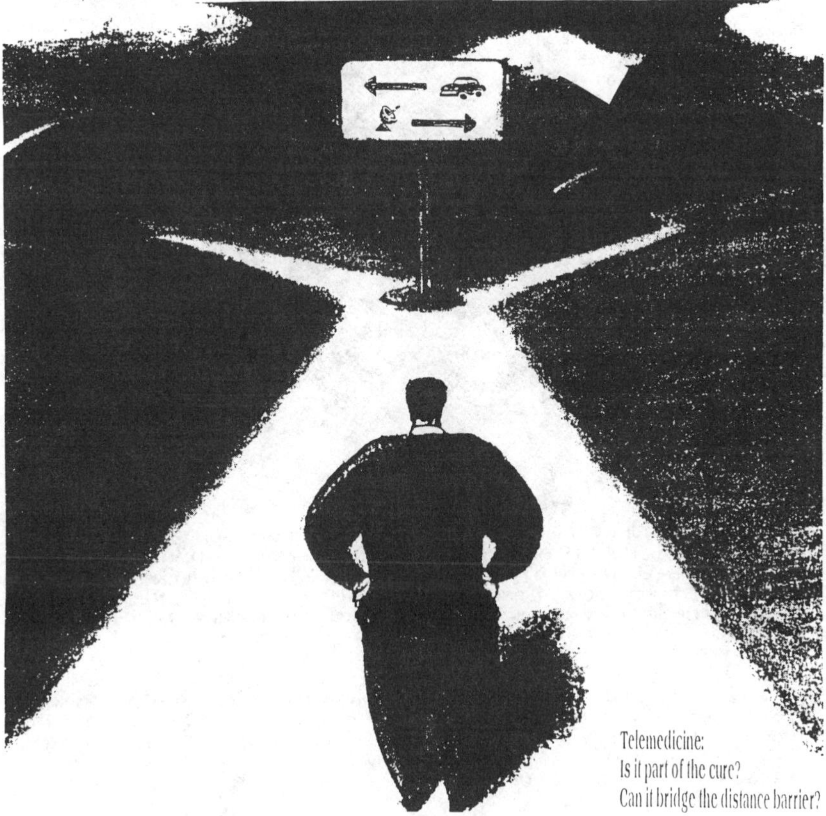

Telemedicine:
Is it part of the cure?
Can it bridge the distance barrier?

THE RURAL TELEMEDICINE WORKSHOP · "Bridging the Distance Barrier" ·November 3-5, 1993 ·Participants List · Ace Allen, M.D., University of Kansas Medical Center · Graham Atkinson, D. Phil. Washington, DC · David C. Balch, East Carolina University School of Medicine · Rashid L. Bashshur, Ph.D., University of Michigan · Laurence H. Beck, Geisinger Health Systems · Peter G. Beeson, Ph.D., Nebraska Department of Public Institutions · Katy Benjamin, Agency for Health Care Policy and Research ·Joseph Binder Rural Electrification Administration · Betsey B. Blakeslee, Ph.D., Center for the New West · James E. Brick, M.D., West Virginia University School of Medicine· Catherine Britain, RODEO NET · Diane D. Brown, SPRINT · Frank Brown, M.D., Emory University · Michael Brown, Cognitive Training Associates, Inc. · Michael S. Brown, Granada Hospital Group · Mark D. Brownell, Office of Congressman Larry LaRocco ·Kathleen Buto, Health Care Financing Administration · Jean Campbell, Ph.D., Maine Department of Mental Health and Mental Retardation ·Daniel W. Campion, Alpha Center · Armand Checker, National Institute of Mental Health · Gerald S. Cohen, Agency for Health Care Policy and Research · Julia A. Cohen, Health Care Financing Administration · Robert D. Colligan, Physicians Practice Group · Steve J. Cotton, Texas Tech HealthNet · Robert M. D'Alessandri, M.D., West Virginia University School of Medicine · Yadin B. David, Ed.D., Texas Children's Hospital · Ruth E. Dayhoff, M.D., Department of Veterans Affairs · Patty Deutsche, Office of Senator Conrad Burns · Jeffrey M. Dunbar, Emory University · Lee Elliott, Office of Representative Glenn English ·Sherry Emery, University of North Carolina · Representative Glenn English, U.S. House of Representatives·Elisa J. Enison, Department of Veterans Affairs · Earl W. Ferguson, M.D., Ph.D., NASA · Frank E. Ferrante, MITRE Corporation · Robert J. Flaherty, M.D., Montana State University · William Fogarty, American Medical Association · Anne Francoeur-Wilson, Health Care Financing Administration · Sherrilynne Fuller, Ph.D., University of Washington · Jack M. Geller, Ph.D., University of North Dakota Center for Rural Health · Elise Gemeinhardt, Office of Senator Alan Simpson · Francoise Gilbert, Altheimer & Gray · Robert E. Gold, M.D., University of Tennessee Medical Group · Cephas L. Goldman, D.D.S., Bureau of Primary Health Care · Millicent Gorham, National Rural Health Association · Arlene Granderson, Office of Rural Health Policy · Jim Grigsby, Ph.D., Center For Health Policy Research· Susan Gustke, M.D., East Carolina University School of Medicine · Allie M. Hanson, Seattle SPRINT · J. Ted Hartman, M.D., Blue Cross/Blue Shield of Texas · Barbara Harvey, Blue Cross/Blue Shield of Texas · W. David Helms, Ph.D., Alpha Center · Colleen Hennessy, Office of Rural Health Policy ·Sheryl D. Hill, US West Communications · Frank T. Hirai, Dartmouth Medical School · Sheri A. Hostetler, Telemedicine Newsletter · A.M. House, M.D., Memorial University of Newfoundland, · Heather E. Hudson, Ph.D., J.D., University of San Francisco · Michael A. Hupfer, Health Care Financing Administration · Linda M. Jacknowitz, West Virginia University · Shirley L. Johnson, Bureau of Health Professions · George H. Kamp, M.D., American College of

Forward

The rural health care system has followed a bumpy road. It has often failed to provide adequate access to health care for the people it serves. Too few primary care practitioners and the need to travel long distances for specialty care have made it difficult for many rural residents to receive the care they need when they need it.

One tool for improving the road to rural health care is telemedicine. Modern telecommunications technology provides an opportunity to improve access to primary and specialty care for rural residents. For example, it is now technologically possible for rural patients to have consultations with distant specialists without leaving their communities.

As is often the case, however, technological capabilities have outpaced the ability of providers to position themselves for its use. In addition, the rate of technologic progress has surpassed policymakers' ability to address regulatory and payment issues that affect the development of rural telemedicine systems. Resolution of these issues must occur before we can tap telemedicine's full potential.

To spur dialogue on these issues, the Office of Rural Health Policy sponsored The Rural Telemedicine Workshop of November 3-5, 1993 in Washington, D.C. Supplemental support for the workshop was provided by the Office of Rural Mental Health Research, National Institute of Mental Health, National Institutes of Health.

This report summarizes the policy issues examined at the workshop and presents options for resolving those issues. We welcome your comments on this report, as well as your thoughts on the problems and opportunities telemedicine presents for rural health care. At the Office of Rural Health Policy, your comments can be directed to Dena Puskin, Cathy Wasem, or Carole Mintzer at 301-443-0835. Our fax number is 301-443-2803. We also can be reached over the internet: dpuskin, cwasem, or cmintzer — @hrsa.ssw.dhhs.gov

Dena S. Puskin, Sc.D.
Deputy Director
Office of Rural Health Policy

Introduction

Rural residents have always faced difficulties in obtaining health care. They often must travel long distances, perhaps missing time from work, to receive care from distant medical centers. Sometimes they do without the care they need. Medical specialists are particularly scarce in rural areas. Many practitioners who serve small communities often miss the professional interaction found in larger medical centers and are driven back to the cities for this reason. Some rural areas face a constant struggle in recruiting and retaining practitioners.

As this nation debates health care reform and struggles to find ways to provide health care more equitably to its citizens, the needs of rural residents and other underserved citizens have been thrust into the spotlight. It is no longer tolerable, assert many medical ethicists and policy makers, that citizens are disqualified from receiving quality health care by virtue of their economic or social status or their geographic location. If this nation is to make meaningful changes in its health care system, it must find innovative ways to surmount the barriers that traditionally have limited access for many of its citizens.

This challenge comes at a time when advances in telecommunications make linking rural and urban communities easier than ever before. In this modern information era, many experts believe that telecommunications could hold the key for providing comprehensive, coordinated health care to rural residents. Electronically-mediated linkages between rural and urban practitioners could not only improve the range and quality of medical services available to rural residents, but alleviate the isolation of rural health care professionals.

The potential of telecommunications to address the needs of rural residents and practitioners is enormous. Applications range from the simple use of the telephone for data transmission to full-motion, two-way interactive video for medical consultation. Rural health practitioners can now conduct consultations in "real time" with specialists in distant medical centers using interactive audio/visual links. This enables rural patients to stay close to home and improves their access to specialty care. Telecommunication systems help reduce professional isolation by providing opportunities for continuing medical education close to home, without the cost and inconvenience of traveling great distances. Telemedicine also can benefit urban practitioners by providing them with a window to the challenges of rural practice and the needs of rural patients. It also facilitates the training of health professional students in rural communities and increases the likelihood they will practice there after graduation.

In recent years, the number of telemedicine projects has expanded rapidly. They include the HealthNet project in west Texas created by the

Texas Tech University Health Sciences Center in Lubbock, the Telemedicine System at the Medical College of Georgia in Augusta, the Eastern Montana Telemedicine Project at Deaconess Medical Center in Billings, the telemedicine program at Kansas University Medical Center in Kansas City, the Rodeo Net Project in eastern Oregon, and the Mountaineer Doctor Television project at West Virginia University in Morgantown.

Given such pioneering, the development of telemedicine is now at a significant juncture. Although telemedicine can bridge the distance barrier from a technological standpoint, it is still considered experimental in many respects. Few studies have examined telemedicine's clinical effectiveness, its acceptability to patients and physicians, its costs, or its ability to reduce practitioner isolation and promote health care networks. There is an overwhelming need for studies that will evaluate telemedicine scientifically and provide meaningful information for future investments. Attention must also be given to the long-term operation and sustainability of telemedicine networks, since most start-up grants are limited in duration. While most experts would agree that telemedicine could radically change the face of rural medicine, the challenge lies in evaluating it and applying it judiciously.

Experts also warn of the costs of not addressing the barriers to health care in rural areas. If innovative strategies are not implemented, the disparity between the urban "haves" and the rural "have nots" may well grow larger.

For telemedicine to realize its potential in rural areas, policy makers must identify and address the barriers to its use. Some federal and state policies obstruct the development of telemedicine networks in communities that could benefit from them. Changes in communications regulations, tariff laws, and medical licensing requirements would facilitate the development of telemedicine networks, as would an increased willingness on the part of insurers to pay for telemedicine consultations.

To address these issues, federal and state policy makers, telecommunications experts, and rural health experts gathered at The Rural Telemedicine Workshop on November 3-5, 1993 in Washington, D.C.. The workshop was sponsored by the federal Office of Rural Health Policy with supplemental support from the Office of Rural Mental Health Research, National Institute of Mental Health. Workshop participants examined the role of telemedicine systems in rural health care network development, identified the key policy issues that affect the implementation of these systems, and proposed policy options to address these issues. This report provides a summary of the workshop discussions and the proposals they helped generate.

"For telemedicine to realize its potential in rural areas, policy makers must identify and address the barriers to its use."

Infrastructure

Infrastructure Development

Telecommunication and information technologies are playing an increasingly important role in business and health. The technology is available, costs are dropping dramatically, and quality is improving. It's ironic then, that the regulatory structure that once ensured equal access to telecommunications is coming apart, says Dena Puskin, ScD, deputy director of the federal Office of Rural Health Policy. The system of subsidies that once supported rural areas has been undermined by the breakup of the Bell System and the shift toward deregulated services. Regulators are calling for fair competition when it is greater collaboration that would better serve rural areas, Puskin says.

Telecommunication regulations are among the greatest obstacles to bringing telemedicine to rural regions. Boundaries of local telephone service areas, established during the breakup of the Bell System, have been a major deterrent in a number of areas. In some regions, telephone calls made to sites within the same local telephone service area can be more expensive than calls made to sites outside these boundaries that are handled by long distance carriers such as AT&T, Sprint, or MCI. For example, in 1992, the Texas MedNet project faced monthly transmission charges within the same local telephone service area of $27 per mile, while the monthly cost of transmission between service areas was $5 per mile. Consequently, telecommunication between a rural and urban hospital within the same local telephone service area can be prohibitively expensive, says Heather Hudson, PhD, JD, director of the Telecommunications Management and Policy Program in the McLaren School of Business at the University of San Francisco.

In most parts of the country, only one local telephone company—either a Bell operating company or an independent company—is allowed to provide service within a local telephone service area. Local telephone rates are regulated by the public utility commission in each state and competition is generally not a factor in keeping rates down. Long distance carriers are currently pressing for regulatory changes that would allow them to compete in the local markets. However, according to Hudson, it is not clear whether this would ultimately lead to lower rates for rural customers because rural areas are not as likely to attract competition.

In short, the costs of transmission, must be lowered if telemedicine is to become economically feasible for many rural hospitals. Telephone rates traditionally have been based on distance, so rural residents have paid higher rates for service. Some analysts have proposed establishing an essential service rate for rural health and social services that would be insensitive to distance, says Sherry Emery, former analyst for the Office of Technology Assessment and a doctoral student at the University of North

Carolina. A minimum level of technological sophistication would be available to all essential service customers. This would allow local governments, hospitals, and educational providers to have access to at least a basic level of service at guaranteed, distance-insensitive prices.

"Phone charges should be distance insensitive for essential services, like health care."

Several policy options that would establish this essential service pricing package have been proposed, Emery says. The government could mandate a flat rate for the service. Or, in areas where there is more than one telecommunications provider, they could bid for that flat rate business. Finally, the boundary of the local telephone service area could be eliminated for essential services.

In addition to addressing pricing issues, workshop participants concluded that an effective national strategic plan for the implementation of telemedicine technologies must foster connectivity and flexibility. State regulatory agencies that establish telecommunications rates can help achieve connectivity by setting standards and protocols that ensure compatibility among communications systems. Such standards already exist within the telephone industry, yet it is important that providers of newer types of communication services, such as cable television and interactive video, also adopt standards, Hudson says. It is also important to ensure that equipment meets the standards that are set. This would ensure that local systems can interconnect and communicate within a national network.

To facilitate the implementation of telemedicine in rural areas, national policies should encourage telephone companies to provide more service flexibility. In particular, workshop participants identified the need for bandwidth-on-demand, an arrangement through which telemedicine providers access and pay for only as much transmission capacity as they need. For example, the transmission of interactive video applications requires high bandwidths, whereas the transmission of less demanding applications, such as EKG's, can be achieved through smaller conduits. Rather than paying for dedicated capacity which often lays dormant, a hospital or clinic could dial up the appropriate amount of bandwidth as needed, and pay for only what it uses.

Workshop participants also identified the need for shared arrangements of telecommunications systems. Providers of telemedicine need to explore ways to share the system with other providers of community services—such as schools, government and social services—as a means to share costs and help meet the other essential needs of rural residents.

Finally, flexibility could be improved by identifying unused communications capacity and applying it to the needs of the community. Some rural communities have vast amounts of buried cable but do not know it exists there. Along with the telephone companies, state lotteries, electric and gas

"Workshop participants strongly recommended that providers at both ends of the teleconsultation receive appropriate payment for their services."

utilities, cable companies, and rural businesses also have a lot of buried fiber and communications capacity that is virtually unknown to other users.

It is very important that states inventory this "dark fiber" and free up surplus capacity. According to Hudson, efforts to utilize dark fiber have been hindered because some local telephone companies do not know how to offer access to this surplus capacity and still comply with state tariff regulations. This is because regulators impose accounting requirements on local telephone companies that inhibit the use of unused capacity.

Some states are considering proposals that would facilitate the usage of surplus capacity, Hudson says. These proposals include waiving the accounting rules or allowing special discount rates for public service applications such as health and education. Many states are giving the telephone companies more flexibility in setting their own rates, often in exchange for commitments to operate more efficiently or to upgrade their networks.

Payment Issues

Payment Issues

Whether or not telemedicine successfully penetrates into many rural areas will depend largely on how payment issues are resolved. Which health care services should be covered and who should be paid? How should its price be determined? Should its price reflect its potential benefits to society, such as lowering professional isolation and improving access to health care? Should transmission and operating costs be covered in addition to professional fees? And who should pay for the equipment?

The Health Care Financing Administration's (HCFA's) willingness to pay for telemedicine services under Medicare is at the heart of the discussions on payment policy. This is because HCFA's approach is often a useful indicator of how other payers will respond. Even after health care reform is passed into law, Medicare is expected to remain a model for payment policies.

Payment for telemedicine is complicated by the diversity of services that can be provided through this technology. Most, however, fall under two broad categories—those that do not involve any direct interaction with a patient, which Medicare currently covers, and those that involve an electronically-mediated interaction with the patient, which Medicare currently does not cover.

Services that do not involve direct patient interaction include the interpretation of radiology tests, pathology slides, or EKGs transmitted electronically to a specialist at a remote site. Medicare pays the same standard fees for these services that it would without electronic transmission, and it makes no additional payment to cover the costs of transmission.

Medicare currently does not pay for electronically-mediated consultations with the patient. This includes interactive consultations in which a primary care practitioner and a specialist present and discuss a patient by interactive video. Medicare also does not consider the use of interactive video as meeting its requirements for physician supervision of physician assistants. In general, Medicare will not cover an electronically-mediated interaction when it replaces direct, face-to-face contact. To date, the only exception is in Georgia, where Medicare, Medicaid, and Blue Cross/Blue Shield pay both the consulting and the referring physician for electronically-mediated consultations, provided that the referring physician is present during the consultation.

Medicare payment for video consultations is one of the most important payment issues in telemedicine today. Those who argue against payment say that video consultations—whether they are held between physicians or between a physician and a patient—are analogous to telephone consultations, which Medicare does not cover. It is presumed that specialists are paid for telephone consultations in the form of resulting referrals.

Graham Atkinson, DPhil, a private consultant specializing in the design of innovative health care payment systems, agrees that video consultations that simply replace telephone conversations should not be reimbursed. "But," he says, "to the extent the video consultation substitutes for a face-to-face visit that would be paid for, and simply saves the patient time and expense in traveling to see the physician, it would seem fair that the physician should be paid for the service provided. The payment in this situation should be the same as if the service were provided conventionally."

Workshop participants strongly recommended that providers at both ends of the teleconsultation receive appropriate payment for their services. For the specialist, it was felt that the appropriate payment in most cases would equal the amount received for traditional consultations. For the primary care practitioner, payment would depend upon the level of involvement in the consultation. The involvement could range from observing and taking a passive role, for which no fee might be appropriate, to actually performing a procedure under the guidance of the specialist, for which a procedure fee might be appropriate. The participants felt that changes in the billing codes may be required to reflect these degrees of participation.

In addition to assigning reasonable prices for telemedicine services, payers need to assess whether telemedicine is safe and effective for all specialty applications. They also need to determine the level of documentation necessary to assure that the service was provided appropriately.

Another payment issue is how to pay for the technical component of tele-

medicine—the capital equipment, overhead and operating costs. Several payment methods have been proposed, Atkinson says. A prospective payment system would establish a payment rate up front, using some sort of fee schedule. Reasonable allowances for the technical costs could be based on the costs incurred by established telemedicine demonstration projects. Alternatively, a cost-based system could be developed to reimburse for actual incurred costs on an ongoing basis. A final option would be to make no payment for the technical component, based on the assumption that payment for professional services alone would likely ensure the dissemination of the technology. The exception to this would be the small rural facility that lacks the financial resources to install or maintain a telemedicine system. Workshop participants proposed that these "essential community providers" receive federal cost-based reimbursement for up to five years to cover the technical expenses of a telemedicine system.

Rural health care providers may want to consider sharing communications facilities with other users, such as the school system, social service organizations, and the local government. Shared arrangements could lower the costs for the technical component borne by the health care system, but also could complicate efforts to allocate expenses and time on the system fairly.

It is not likely that video consultations will disseminate to many rural communities without changes in the payment system. Workshop participants at the telemedicine workshop called for statutory and regulatory changes to payment policy that recognize the potential benefit of telemedicine to rural America. Such policies could breathe new life into struggling rural communities, especially those with troubled hospitals. Rural patients will seek treatment closer to home when they know that specialists are "on site" through telemedicine. Telemedicine may also strengthen rural health systems by reducing professional isolation, providing rural training opportunities for health professional students, and making it easier to recruit and retain health care professionals.

Legal Aspects

Legal Aspects

The problem of malpractice liability is potentially a great obstacle to the general application of telemedicine, says Jonathan Sanders, JD, former associate with Weil, Gotshal & Manges, New York, NY, and a medical student. Although there has been little evidence of telemedicine-related malpractice litigation, it is likely that the legal profession will focus greater attention on this area as medical centers with "deep pockets" form telemedicine networks.

By its very nature, telemedicine may inherently expose practitioners to malpractice claims, says Sanders. The public may perceive that a telemedicine consultation is somehow inadequate because it does not involve a "hands on" examination. In addition, misconceptions about digital compression technology could influence the outcome of malpractice cases. Although the process of digital compression eliminates only the information that is repetitious from one frame to the next, a jury might conclude that the consulting physician worked with incomplete data. However, several quality assurance studies have demonstrated that images constructed from digitally compressed signals are adequate. For example, in a study of thirty patients with dermatologic problems conducted by the Medical College of Georgia, researchers found no difference between the diagnoses made using a telecommunication link and those made in person.

"Several steps could be taken to limit liability."

Several steps could be taken to limit liability. National health professional associations (eg, the American College of Radiology, the American College of Cardiology, and the College of Dermatology) could establish technical standards for the quality of transmission and images needed for various applications. Consulting physicians could limit their liability by ensuring that their technical systems meet these standards and by declining to make a diagnostic interpretation if these standards are not met. Also, physicians may want to videotape the entire consultation—as a record-keeping measure and as documentation for liability purposes. Finally, Sanders says, physicians and medical centers that provide telemedicine consultations to the underserved could be protected from lawsuits under the doctrine of "sovereign immunity." This could take the form of a cap on economic damages or some other hold-harmless protection.

The potential to electronically transfer a patient's medical records raises important issues of confidentiality and the patient's right to privacy. How does one ensure that personal and sensitive medical records do not become available to others who would use them inappropriately? Clear, simple and comprehensive policies are needed to protect medical records when they are transmitted and stored, says Françoise Gilbert, Esq, chair of the Information Technology Division of the American Bar Association and partner with Altheimer & Gray in Chicago. Such policies should encompass the management and use of patient records, as well as physical security measures and the protection of software, hardware and telecommunication tools, she says.

Large, complex computer systems installed at health care facilities are vulnerable to many types of threats that could lead to the destruction, modification, or inappropriate use of patient medical records, Gilbert says. Computer viruses and malicious attacks by computer hackers, disgruntled personnel or vendors threaten the security of electronic records and could result in large liability. Health care providers remain responsible for implementing a reasonable level of security for their computer systems, including their electronic patient records systems, Gilbert says.

Data processing or telecommunication disasters also are prone to occur, Gilbert says, and providers and clinics that rely heavily on computers or telecommunications must implement sufficient back-up of these systems. Health care providers also can be found negligent if they fail to back up their systems and a patient's care is interrupted because their electronic medical records cannot be accessed.

Licensure

Licensure

The state licensure system effectively requires a physician practicing telemedicine to be licensed in every state in which he or she practices. Such a system places a great a burden on physicians wishing to provide telemedicine consultations to citizens residing across state lines.

Several changes to the state licensing system have been proposed, says Jay H. Sanders, MD, professor of medicine and director of the Telemedicine Center at the Medical College of Georgia in Augusta. First, individual state licensure for telemedicine could be converted to a national health care licensure system similar to the military. Second, for specialty consultations, the referring physician could retain responsibility for the patient's care, so that any "care" provided by a physician in another state could be viewed as a recommendation only. Third, and perhaps the simplest way to deal with state licensure, is to consider the patient as being "electronically transported" to the physician rather than the physician being transported to the patient.

Finally, telemedicine consultations conducted across state lines are a form of interstate commerce and could become the concern of the Federal Trade Commission. So far, the commission has not concerned itself with telemedicine or imposed additional regulatory and licensing requirements.

Effects

Effects on Health Care Costs

The overall impact of telemedicine on health care costs is unclear. Moreover, Puskin cautions, the measure of success for telemedicine should not be whether it saves money, but whether it improves access to care for underserved populations at a reasonable price.

Telemedicine proponents believe that substantial savings can be realized by providing quality health care in the rural setting and reducing visits to more costly urban centers. On the other hand, with improved access to care, formerly underserved populations can be expected to use more care and drive up total health care expenditures.

From the standpoint of third-party payers, telemedicine may not save costs. Karl Katterjohn, vice president of Med-Scene, points out that the balance sheet is further complicated because many of the savings realized through telemedicine are of value to society but are not factored in as reimbursable costs under the current payment system. These benefits include more preventive care, lower transportation costs, and less time lost from work.

"It is the social benefits from telemedicine that are so difficult to measure."

Researchers are just beginning to evaluate the cost savings from telemedicine. According to Jay Sanders, MD, preliminary data from the telemedicine project at the Medical College of Georgia indicates that 81% of the patients who receive care through telemedicine have not required transfers to secondary or tertiary care centers. Given that the average cost of a bed per day at Dodge County Hospital in rural Eastman, GA, is $800, compared to $1300 at the Medical College of Georgia in Augusta, the findings suggest that substantial savings could be made by providing quality health care through the rural hospital. Because the costs at Dodge County Hospital are typical of rural hospitals in Georgia, the study's authors estimate that an increase of a single patient per day to the rural hospital census represents a net cash flow of $150,000 per year for the hospital. This is revenue that is staying in the rural community, enhancing not only the fiscal stability of the rural hospital but also the socioeconomic fabric of the community, Sanders says. Additional data from more telemedicine projects will have to be collected to determine whether this preliminary evidence of savings can be substantiated.

Telemedicine also can bring revenue into the rural community by facilitating the more rapid "repatriation" of rural residents discharged from distant tertiary care centers. Providers in tertiary care centers who can follow-up their rural patients' care through telecommunications might discharge them sooner than they would if this option were not available.

Telemedicine can further cut health care costs by facilitating the treatment of patients at an earlier stage of their disease process and by transmitting education programs on disease prevention to the community. Both of these benefits can potentially cut long-term costs by decreasing hospitalization stays and increasing productivity. Furthermore, bridging the distance barrier electronically saves the costs of transporting medical personnel and equipment.

It is the social benefits from telemedicine, which are so difficult to measure, that make cost-effectiveness analysis a minefield for guiding decision making on telemedicine. Cost-effectiveness analysis requires precise specifications of the inputs and outcomes of the systems being measured. However, improved access and quality, benefits from preventive care, and rural economic development are difficult to quantify and are likely to be left

Acceptance

"... telemedicine systems must be simple to use and tailor-made for specific needs."

out of the cost-effectiveness equation. When this occurs, the cost-effectiveness analysis will misrepresent telemedicine's true benefits and lead to sub-optimal decisions on whether and how to invest in these systems.

Acceptability to Practitioners and Patients

The medical community has become increasingly interested in applying telecommunication systems to rural health care. Many perceive telemedicine to be a potentially important tool for providing a comprehensive, coordinated system of health care to rural residents. By creating linkages between professional colleagues, telemedicine systems could improve the range and quality of medical services available to rural residents while alleviating some of the professional isolation experienced by rural practitioners.

Several factors could account for these positive views. Equipment and transmission costs have fallen dramatically. Health professionals have become more comfortable using computers and telecommunications technologies in general. And the advent of digital compression has brought the technology to a point where it can meet most clinical requirements for transmission and resolution.

Twenty years ago, video images were transmitted using costly analog signals. Today, an analog image can be converted into a digital signal, transmitted, and converted back into an analog image at the receiving site. The resolution for analog and digital signals is comparable. However, digital systems can transmit sound, pictures, and data simultaneously, thus using telecommunications capacity more efficiently. Digital signals also can carry more information at a lower cost than analog. Digitally-compressed images can have a resolution nearly rivaling that of television, making them suitable for many clinical applications. Furthermore, improvements in technology have been coupled with dramatic reductions in costs, so that what was once only feasible for large, well-financed medical centers has become an option for an increasing number of rural hospitals.

The workshop participants emphasized that telemedicine systems must be simple to use and tailor-made for specific needs. Community leaders should be involved in identifying these needs. And because each medical specialty requires different technical capabilities, telemedicine systems must be designed with the intended application in mind. Radiologists and pathologists, for example, require high resolution images for interpretation and diagnosis, yet rehabilitation specialists may find lower resolution sufficient for analyzing movement. Mental health professionals may prefer a system that their patients can use directly, without a technician in the room. And cardiologists may need an electronic stethoscope with high quality audio and "real time" transmission of echocardiograms.

National health professional associations should be leaders in setting standards for transmission and fidelity for the telemedicine applications within their specialties. Such standards would ensure practitioners that the information and images they receive through telecommunications are of the quality necessary for their intended applications. Adherence to standards also would limit health professional liability.

Ultimately, the value of telemedicine rests with how the patients perceive and adapt to it, says Sanders. Patients are not likely to accept telemedicine consultations if they perceive them as being too impersonal or costly, or if they want their practitioner physically by their side. Previous telemedicine projects have found that patients are more likely to accept systems that are easy to use, allow direct eye contact, and give them control of the interview camera. Some patients have reported feeling that they were being treated in a very special way. Much more research is needed to determine how patients and health professionals respond to telemedicine.

"In the final analysis, it will be the human touch at each end of the system—not the technology—that will determine whether it is successful or not," Sanders predicts.

"It will be the human touch at each end of the system that will determine its success."

Conclusion

Unlike the interstate highway, the goal of the electronic highway is to move information rather than people. However, just as the interstates bypassed many rural communities, contributing to their economic decline, there is a risk that the same could happen with the infrastructure for the electronic highway. Although telecommunications has tremendous potential to aid the economic development of rural communities, without adequate infrastructure, that potential will not be realized.

Similarly, telemedicine holds promise as a tool for improving the rural health care system, but will require adequate telecommunications and human infrastructures to be effective. Telemedicine can foster the growth of integrated health care systems that serve both rural patients and rural providers. It provides rural patients with access to comprehensive health care services, both in their community and from distant providers. And rural practitioners would find their practice less isolating because telemedicine facilitates frequent contact with distant colleagues who share their interests. Such interactions would simulate the professional associations that are commonplace in urban areas.

At this point in time, however, health care providers who are contemplating involvement in telemedicine systems face the obstacles described in this report. They look at the technology in the context of health care delivery and discover that policymakers and regulators have not shaped tariffs, payment policies, and laws that respond to the pace of technological progress and its applications for health care. Each provider also looks for information about costs, acceptability, appropriateness, and quality, but finds few answers.

Yet, much like telephones today, the day will come when telemedicine is fully integrated into the rural health care system. Scientific evaluations will have been conducted and the regulatory and payment issues will have been resolved. Many actors will have participated in this process including the federal government, Congress, states, telephone companies, health care providers and other public and private entities.

The time has arrived for all these players to respond to the opportunities at hand and make telecommunications technology the good servant of rural health care. In so doing, all involved are responsible for ensuring that telemedicine improves access to health care for rural residents and enhances the professional life of rural practitioners at an affordable price.

"The time has arrived to respond to the opportunities at hand and assure that rural communities are not bypassed by the electronic highway."

Author
Teri Randall

Chief Editor
Carole Mintzer

Associate Editors
Dena Puskin
Cathy Wasem
Sue Bernstein
Alice Adams

Cover Photo
© 1994 Laura Tedschi
Stock Illustration Source

Special Photo Credits and Thanks to
Lumiere Studios, © George Cannon
Inside Front Cover

Texas Tech University Health Sciences Center/HealthNet,
Pages 2, 4, 8, 11, 13 and 15

West Virginia University
Pages 7 and Inside Back Cover

For more information, contact the
Federal Office of Rural Health Policy
5600 Fishers Lane, Room 9-05
Rockville, MD 20857
(301) 443-0835

Radiology · Andrew Krackov, U.S. News and World Report · Karl Katterjohn, P.A., MedScene · Barbara Kerlin, Ph.D., MITRE Corporation · Henry B. King, Ph.D., Appalachian Regional Commission · Keith R. Krueger, Friends of the National Library of Medicine · K. Sue Kwentus, R.N., Onancock, VA · Su-san Lancoon, Office of Congressman Amory Houghton · Linda J. Laskowski, US West Communications · Jim K. Long, West River Regional Medical Center · Fabia Mahoney, The Bureau of National Affairs · Louis Emmet Mahoney, M.D., Health Resources and Services Administration · Paul Maakestad, Mercy Foundation · James S. Martin, Mayo Clinic · William T. McCaughan, Ed.D., Texas Tech HealthNet · Harriet G. McCombs, Ph.D., Substance Abuse and Mental Health Services Administration · David L. McHugh, MTI Medical Televideo, Inc. · Andrew M. Mekelburg, Bell Atlantic Network Services, Inc.· Lynn L. Merritt-Nixon, Health Care Financing Administration · Robin Meter, University of Nebraska Medical Center · Carole L. Mintzer, Office of Rural Health Policy · Richard Morrissey, Kansas Department of Health and Environment · Lawrence D. Nadel, Ph.D., MITRE Corporation · Craig D. Obey, J.D., Office of Senator Kent Conrad · John C. Oeffinger, Texas Hospital Education & Research Foundation · Douglas C. Overlock, Eastern Oregon Human Services Consortium · Kevin Patrick, Office of Disease Prevention-Health Promotion/PHS · Daniel Pearson, Committee on Science, Space and Technology · Fred Peralta, Carle Foundation · Douglas A. Perednia, M.D., Oregon Health Sciences University · Bonnie D. Post, Maine Ambulatory Care Coalition · Jane Preston, M.D., Telemedical Interactive Consultative Services, Inc. · Dena S. Puskin, Sc.D., Office of Rural Health Policy · Neil Rambo, University of Washington · Jim Reid, Deaconess Medical Center · Bernice Reyes-Akinbileje, Congressional Research Service · Cindy Roberts, United States Department of Agriculture · William A. Robinson, M.D., Health Resources and Services Administration · Greg Rohde, Office of Senator Byron Dorgan · Jay H. Sanders, M.D., Medical College of Georgia, · Deborah E. Seale, University of Texas · John P. Seidenberg, Healthcare Telecom Report · Jacqueline L. Sheridan, Health Care Financing Administration · Tina Shoemaker, Rural Health Consultants · Diane J. Skiba, Ph.D., University of Colorado Health Sciences Center · Gregory L. Smith, Solutions Plus, Inc. · Jean E. Smith, Office of Technology Assessment · Glen R. Southworth, Colorado Video Incorporated · Mark P. Steinhorn, Compression Labs, Inc. · Eric Tangalos, M.D., Mayo Foundation Communications Committee · Patricia Taylor, Ph.D., Office of Rural Health Policy · Nancy H. Temple, Carolinas Medical Center · Heidi Thoren, Family Practice News · Dan Trott, Eastman Kodak Company · Leslie A. Tucker, American Academy of Family Physicians · Charles F. Turcan, Telemedical Systems Integration · Cathy Wasem, Office of Rural Health Policy · Sheldon D. Weisgrau, Health Care Financing Administration · Bill M. Welch, Nevada Rural Hospital Project · Charles Windle, Ph.D., Office of Rural Mental Health Research · Patricia F. Wright-Gaines, Health Care Financing Administration · Sarkis M. Zartarian, D.Sc., Apex, NC

RURAL TELEHEALTH:

Telemedicine, Distance Education and Informatics for Rural Health Care

September, 1993

A report of the

Office of Rural Health Policy

Health Resources and Services Administration
Public Health Service
U.S. Department of Health and Human Services

Prepared by the

Western Cooperative for Educational Telecommunications
Western Interstate Commission for Higher Education

RURAL TELEHEALTH:
Telemedicine, Distance Education and Informatics for Rural Health Care

A Report of the
Office of Rural Health Policy
Health Resources and Services Administration, DHHS

Prepared by
Western Cooperative for Educational Telecommunications
Western Interstate Commission for Higher Education
Boulder, Colorado

Written by
John P. Witherspoon
Sally M. Johnstone
Cathy J. Wasem

The Authors

John P. Witherspoon served as the principal author of the report's primer section. He is Professor Emeritus of Telecommunications and Film at San Diego State University, and Director of the Pacific Dialogue, a program addressing communication issues in the development of a Pacific Region community. He has served as the president of the Public Service Satellite Consortium, the first principal executive for television at the Corporation for Public Broadcasting, a public broadcasting manager, and the first Board Chairman of National Public Radio.

Sally M. Johnstone is the Director of the Western Cooperative for Educational Telecommunications, a project of the Western Interstate Commission for Higher Education. Dr. Johnstone has led this membership organization of the 15 western states since is formal inception in 1989. She has also developed and administered educational telecommunications systems in both rural and urban areas, written articles on educational telecommunications applications and policies, consulted at state and institutional levels, and served on college and university psychology faculties.

Cathy J. Wasem is Director of Information Services and Policy Development, federal Office of Rural Health Policy, DHHS. Prior to joining the Office in 1988, she directed the Oglala Lakota College Nursing Program on the Pine Ridge Indian Reservation in South Dakota and a health careers program at Sinte Gleska University on the Rosebud Reservation. She has worked as a staff nurse at a rural Indian Health Service hospital, and for the U.S. Public Health Service Hospital, Seattle, WA. She studied German health policy as a DAAD/Fulbright scholar in Cologne, Germany.

Copies of this report may be obtained, while supplies last, for $8.00 to cover postage and handling from:

WICHE Publications
P.O. Drawer P
Boulder, CO 80301-9752

* Payment must accompany order *

This document was prepared by the Western Cooperative for Educational Telecommunications under purchase order number HRSA 92-1208 (P). Initial research on rural health issues and on health programs using telecommunication technologies was conducted by the Intergovernmental Health Policy Project, George Washington University under purchase order number HRSA 91-871 (P).

Preparation of this report was supported by the Office of Rural Health Policy, Health Resources and Services Administration, Public Health Service, U.S. Department of Health and Human Services, 5600 Fishers Lane, Room 9-05, Rockville, MD 20857. Cathy Wasem of the Office of Rural Health Policy served as project officer.

PREFACE

This document was prepared to assist rural communities considering the use of telecommunication and information technologies in their health care systems. It provides a simple and objective overview of the various technologies available and their rural applications. It also discusses the issues currently affecting the development and use of these technologies in rural areas.

Telecommunication and information technologies hold promise for the overall development of rural communities. Certainly they will play a key role in the development of health care networks under health care reform. They can decrease the isolation of rural health professionals -- promoting their retention and recruitment and even providing a way for rural communities to develop or "grow their own" health professionals. Telecommunication and information technologies can also improve and maintain the quality of care available in small communities by giving rural clinicians access to the latest biomedical information. Finally, such modern technology can enhance the range of the actual health services available locally, thus retaining health care dollars in the community.

Telecommunications can spell power and partnerships for rural communities. To tap its potential, however, local planners need objective information on the opportunities and options available. We hope this publication provides that information. Because the environment changes rapidly, and the number of telecommunications projects in the health field is increasing, the Office of Rural Health Policy has made plans to update this booklet within a year. Suggestions for improvements and revisions are welcome.

Dena S. Puskin, Sc.D.
Acting Director
Office of Rural Health Policy
DHHS

Sally Johnstone, Ph.D.
Director
Western Cooperative for
Educational Telecommunications

TABLE OF CONTENTS

INTRODUCTION:
TELECOMMUNICATION and INFORMATION TECHNOLOGIES AND RURAL HEALTH CARE

Many rural areas have very limited access to health care services. That's hardly news; the problem is to address the issue within the bounds of acceptable cost and available people and technology. The rural situation is not simply a low-population version of urban health care issues. A 1990 study by the Office of Technology Assessment (OTA) cited three problems that are specific to residents of rural areas:

- o Although the rural population has relatively low mortality rates, a disproportionate number of rural people suffer from chronic illnesses. Furthermore, infant mortality is slightly higher than in urban areas and the number of deaths from injury are dramatically higher.

- o The lack of a public transportation system and the existence of few local providers make it difficult for rural individuals to reach facilities where they can obtain care. Individuals living in areas with six or fewer residents per square mile, (i.e., frontier rural areas) have "geographical access problems of immense proportions." Moreover, in such counties there is often an insufficient population base to adequately support local health services.

- o The OTA found that the physical barriers to access -- difficult as they are -- may be outweighed by financial barriers. In 1987 one out of every six rural families lived in poverty, compared to one out of every eight in urban areas. And, rural residents below the federal poverty level were less likely to be covered by Medicaid than urban residents (35.5 v. 44.4 percent).

Increasingly specialized and expensive medical technology and procedures make the access problem worse. The National Governors Association has reported that rural areas have less than half the physician coverage available in urban areas. Moreover, rural hospitals cannot afford to purchase limited use, state of the art technologies. As a result, these small community facilities find it difficult to compete with larger -- if more distant -- medical centers, and they are often forced to close. The U.S. General Accounting Office (GAO) has reported that half the community hospital closings during the 1980s were in rural areas. When those hospitals close, residents in the communities they serve lose an important entry point into the health care system. Meanwhile, many studies suggest that these rural communities may have disproportionately greater needs for health care than their urban and suburban counterparts, particularly in the area of emergency services. It has been estimated, for example, that about 60 percent of traffic fatalities occur in rural areas. In addition, rural residents are more likely to be engaged in hazardous occupations.

81-951 0 - 94 - 7

There have been many initiatives to address these issues of rural access, and an increasing number of them are relying upon telecommunication and information technologies to foster access. Everything from phone and fax to video and high-speed computing has been enlisted to provide specialty services, consultations and continuing education.

This report provides an introduction to the technologies related to telecommunications, and it shows how these technologies are being applied to enhance access to health care for people in rural areas.

A PRIMER OF RELEVANT TELECOMMUNICATION AND INFORMATION TECHNOLOGIES[1]

This section offers an introduction to the principal technologies of telecommunication, pointing out their main characteristics, a bit of history, and some elements of cost.

There are two broad divisions: the media of telecommunication (the telephone, video, computer, etc.) and the means of transmission (phone lines including optical fiber lines, satellites, microwave systems, etc.).

The media -- telephones, video cameras and monitors, fax machines, computers, etc. -- might be considered the input-output devices of the system: we use them to send and receive voices, pictures, text, diagnostic images, and sounds. The means of transmission actually carry the products of these media, i.e., the words, pictures, etc., from sender to receiver.

A note about costs: Firm dollar amounts are not used here because in key areas they change too rapidly for references to be useful over the lifespan of a publication like this. A typical pattern finds prices dropping dramatically as new products and services find acceptance. For example, today's computers are increasingly powerful and relatively cheap because the main elements of computing -- processing and memory -- have had price reductions of about 50 percent every three years for the past 40 years! The result is not only that we do familiar tasks less expensively, but that the underlying technology can be applied in new ways, setting off yet another round of innovation with cost implications rippling in all directions.

In spite of the frantic pace of innovation, however, it is possible to understand the technological menu and make sensible choices.

A preliminary note: While this is certainly not a technical treatise, even the most technophobic among us eventually must confront two key words, used so often that understanding them makes it far easier to follow the menu. They are "bandwidth" and "digital."

[1] For readers new to the terminology of telecommunication and information technologies, a glossary of terms has been developed. It includes terms used in this document, as well as terms readers may come across in future readings on the topic.

1. Bandwidth. Bandwidth is simply a measurement of a telecommunication channel's capacity, "the size of the pipe." The necessary bandwidth varies with the amount of information to be transmitted. For example, an AM radio station located at 600 KHz on your dial actually occupies the band between 595 and 605; it needs a bandwidth of 10 KHz in the electromagnetic spectrum where broadcasting takes place. (KHz means kilohertz, or thousand hertz. A hertz is one wave cycle per second.) A telephone needs only to handle the sound of a voice; it is designed for a bandwidth of four KHz. A television station, transmitting moving pictures as well as sound, needs a bandwidth of six megahertz (6 MHz or 6 million hertz).

Channel capacity -- bandwidth -- is sometimes expressed also as the number of bits (or sets of bits, called bytes) per second that the channel can handle. (A bit is a "unit of information" in a computer-based binary number system.) One might be tempted to assume that each of a television channel's six million wave cycles per second could carry the off-or-on message of one bit, and therefore six megahertz would equal six megabits (six million bits per second or 6Mbps). But in fact there is no fixed relationship between a hertz and a bit. Today a bandwidth of six megahertz commonly carries between three and ten megabits. Digital technology holds both imperatives and opportunities for those who use it to encode information. It will be seen below that some of this coding magic is making possible major economies and efficiencies in the transmission of video.

The important parts of all this are:

- The more information that must be sent (sound, pictures, bits of information) the more bandwidth that is required. Moving images take more bandwidth than still images; color takes more bandwidth than black-and-white.

- Bandwidth costs money. The greater the bandwidth, the higher the cost.

2. Digital and analog. When you turn on your car radio, you hear the result of a process that draws an electronic picture -- makes an electronic analog -- of the frequencies and relative volume of the original sound. If you were to look at that picture on an engineer's oscilloscope, you would see a pattern of wave forms marching across the tube. Morse's telegraph, on the other hand, encoded words through a pattern of clicks formed by switching electric current off and on very rapidly.

Today's digital technology has more in common with Morse's telegraph than with the radio station's electronic wave forms. Digital coding, represented by zeros and ones, is actually an elegantly simple process of encoding information by turning the power off and on. A bit -- a zero or one in the coding scheme -- is simply the presence or absence of a minute amount of power during a very small interval of time.

The world is rapidly moving toward digital systems for everything from telephones to television. The reasons are straightforward:

- o Since digital systems reduce all kinds of information (sound, pictures, data) to off-on bits, it is possible to send different kinds of information simultaneously through the same channel.
- o Digital systems can use transmission channels more efficiently than can analog systems.
- o Digital systems generally reproduce information more accurately, thus providing users with higher quality than analog systems can handle.

There are cost implications in both directions. Since digital systems can use transmission channels more efficiently, transmission costs may go down. But since digital systems can be quite complex, the necessary equipment may be more expensive. One handy example: in order to realize the economies of digital video, one must buy a codec. At the receiving end of the system, a codec converts the incoming digital video signal back to analog so that your analog television set can display it. Codec is a contraction for COde-DECode. A computer modem (MOdulate-DEModulate) performs similar duty in allowing you to send your computer's digital messages via an analog phone line.

On balance, digital technology has much to recommend it in spite of these complexities, and the world is moving strongly toward digital systems.

The implications of these two concepts -- bandwidth and digital/analog -- will become apparent as we consider specific technologies in the sections to follow.

The Media of Telecommunication

The Telephone: An old friend learns to fly

The telephone, patented just 40 years after Morse's telegraph (in 1876) is easily the most important telecommunication device ever created. Sometimes overlooked as a little old-fashioned for today's high-tech telecommunication projects, the telephone has some major advantages:

- o Ubiquity. Virtually everybody has one. Universal telephone service has been a goal of public policy in the United States for 60 years.

- o Relatively low cost. The cost of basic installation has often been covered, the telephone is a narrowband instrument (doesn't use much bandwidth), and training time is minimal even when new applications are envisioned.

- o Cost per-use is low because system costs are spread among an enormous number of users.

The telephone is a lot more than what the industry calls POTS: Plain Old Telephone Service. It can be applied very flexibly because of the range of services which have emerged during the past few years. These include:

- o Conferencing, in which relatively large numbers of people, geographically dispersed, can meet together by phone. A device called a conference bridge makes it possible to interconnect the participants and maintain good technical quality. For those whose conference requirement is infrequent, it is usually best to contract with a conference service for the bridge and operator support.

- o Voicemail, for the transmission of voice messages when instant response is not required. The basic "answering machine" sort of voicemail can be extended to provide mailboxes for project participants or, for example, to send a voicemail message simultaneously to members of a defined group.

- o Fax, for the transmission of material on paper via the telephone system. Initially developed half a century ago, fax has become nearly ubiquitous as the perceived need for the service coincided with the application of cost-saving microelectronics plus the economies of volume manufacturing.

- o Computer communication, which uses the phone system -- and perhaps other networks -- to exchange electronic mail, transmit documents (and an increasing variety of other things), and engage in electronic conferencing. See the next section below.

- o And picturephones, which transmit a picture of those talking, have been a perennial "just around the corner" technology but may be coming closer to everyday use.

Computer Networking: the Number-Cruncher as Communication Device

One of the fastest-growing areas of telecommunication is communication by computer. There are two complementary applications: electronic mail and computer conferencing.

As its name implies, electronic mail allows the user to address a message to another person or to a group. The message is usually in text form, but system advances make it increasingly feasible to send pictures, charts and diagrams, and sound as well. The message is held in the recipient's electronic mailbox -- located in a network node computer, rather like your local branch post office -- until the recipient dials in and collects it.

Computer conferencing uses some of the same techniques as electronic mail, but it can best be described as an online conference in which the participants are not expected to be present at the same time. Conferences are organized by topic. When a participant dials in, he/she can read what colleagues have contributed, then add related comments as appropriate. At first glance the topic-and-reply format may strike one as a bit rigid, but in fact conferences can be organized in many ways and provide a surprisingly personal and flexible means of communication within a group.

Electronic bulletin boards fall somewhere between conferences and electronic mail. Users may read, post or respond to messages on a "bulletin board" organized by topics.

The Internet. For those in education, government, and research, the most common network for computer communication is the Internet, the largest computer network in the world. The Internet is actually a network of networks, involving the National Science Foundation's NSFNet and a huge complex of university system networks and other networks related to research and government. The proposed National Research and Education Network (NREN), currently known as the Interagency Interim National Research and Education Network (IINREN) will vastly increase the size and capability of today's Internet. Because of the federal government's financial investment through the National Science Foundation, there are currently a number of Congressional bills that aim to put into place a national information infrastructure, referred to as NII. NREN related activities would be encompassed by this NII.

In addition to providing major communication capabilities, the Internet is the venue for a huge amount of information stored in accessible databases. At present the use of the Internet appears free to the end user because the costs have been covered by affiliated institutions and the system is organized so that costs are not, like phone charges, usage-sensitive. This may change in the future, however.

Several other networks are available to computer users, including such diverse systems as MCI Mail and the Prodigy service. Not all networks support all services (particularly conferencing), but each has its strength. Most have usage-sensitive pricing, which can quickly discourage database browsing, not to mention online schmoozing.

Audiographics: Multimedia on a Budget

Think of it as an illustrated lecture: the lecturer's voice is transmitted along with quick chalkboard-like sketches, diagrams, etc., to which students can respond either orally or via an electronic sketch pad. The combination is sent via telephone technology. The result is a system that offers the flexibility of voice-plus-visuals at a cost far below that of most video-based systems. Furthermore, these systems are becoming much more powerful and flexible as the graphic capabilities of computers are brought to bear. In a typical application, a course or meeting conducted from a central location involves participants at one or several remote sites.

Video: Ringside at the Revolution

For many of its pioneers (from not so many years ago) today's video technology must be scarcely recognizable. The pictures we see at home haven't changed much for most people, but the underlying technology is in the midst of a revolution, with significant implications for users such as the health care system, education, and business. Following are some of the important variations.

Full-motion "broadcast" video. This is the video you usually see when you turn on the set at home. There's an enormous amount of information in every frame: in the U.S., 525 lines of video are scanned 30 times a second to reproduce the colors, brightness, and motion of the original. The result consumes an impressive amount of bandwidth: each television station in the U.S. is allotted six MHz (the bandwidth allocated for all the FM stations on your dial would accommodate only three television stations). When this broadcast-standard video is networked by satellite it commands a significant share of the satellite's total capacity. As noted above, bandwidth is expensive.

Compressed video. A major development of the 1980s was the marriage of telecommunication and computing. One result was the application of digital technology to video. That makes it possible to take a fresh look at how video pictures are made. No longer is it necessary to scan every colored dot of all 525 lines 30 times a second in order to make a picture. Using digital technology it is possible to send only those portions of the picture which change frame-to-frame, plus a code that tells the system "Play it again, Sam" for those portions of the picture that don't change. Furthermore, not every application requires 30 frames per second in order to have useful video. The resulting efficiencies can be dramatic. While a conventional six MHz television signal commonly has been translated to a digital format of approximately 45 megabits per second (45Mbps), compressed video for telemedicine consultations is being transmitted at 1.544 Mbps (and in some cases even lower). Compressed video for some business and educational applications is being transmitted at 56 kilobits per second (56 thousand bits versus 45 million bits!).

So while the initial cost of the digital technology is higher than for conventional analog video, the bandwidth requirement is much less, which means that transmission costs can be reduced dramatically. For many applications, video of good quality becomes affordable.

As further advances are made in compression technology, we can expect video of good quality to require even less bandwidth. For many applications we already see video transmitted over lines the phone companies have labeled T1. A T1 line has a bandwidth of 1.544 Mbps; i.e., it can transmit 1.544 megabits per second. The key lesson is that one should no longer assume that video is too expensive.

<u>Interactive video</u>. Given the economies of compressed video, plus the smaller, less expensive video equipment now available, it is now common to have two-way video links for teleconferences, education, and comparable applications. Participants at multiple sites can see and hear each other during the event. Costs for such a service can be very attractive. In the Oregon ED-NET system, for example, multi-site interactive video has an hourly transmission cost that is approximately one-fifth that of one-way "conventional" broadcast-standard video.

Interaction doesn't necessarily imply two-way video. Some systems are based on one-way video with voice return (often by telephone), or a return channel that carries information from a keypad, computer, graphics tablet, etc. This technology can be expected to evolve rapidly and cost less as it is applied to such consumer applications as interactive game shows, shopping channels, etc.

<u>Slow-scan video</u>. Slow-scan, or still-picture video is a method of providing transmission of still pictures over conventional phone lines. As demonstrated above, motion needs substantial bandwidth, and for many applications the cost of that much bandwidth is unacceptable and/or transmission of motion is not necessary. Slow-scan video trades bandwidth for time: it can yield good picture quality over an ordinary phone line by stretching out the time it takes to send the information. Rather than 30 frames of moving video per second, a slow-scan system may take several seconds to more than a minute for a single frame, depending on the quality desired. Slow-scan video has been used successfully for

transmission of X-ray images and other diagnostic imaging, using ordinary twisted-pair copper phone lines and the bandwidth of an ordinary phone call.

A variation of slow-scan video provides computer-to-computer transmission of similar images.

The Means of Transmission

Introduction

In designing a telecommunication system for rural health care or comparable specialized applications, the basic questions are:

- How many sites must be reached?
- Where are they? How far from the "headquarters" location and from each other?
- What potentially useful facilities already exist, e.g. telephone lines, cable TV, satellite send/receive facilities, microwave systems, fiber optic trunks for cable TV or telephone, or a private or government carrier?
- What is the nature of the information to be transmitted: video, audio, computer data, etc.? What are the givens concerning media and equipment to be used (existing video studios, computer facilities, etc.)?
- How much information is to be transmitted at a given time (i.e. what is the bandwidth requirement?)
- How much interaction is required, and where are those who must interact?
- What are the practical financial limitations? What are the priorities separating "must have" from "nice to have"?
- How long is the project intended to last?

Answers to these questions lead to tradeoffs about the technologies to be applied.

The Telephone Network (AKA the Public Switched Telephone Network - PSTN)

The world's fundamental telecommunications network is the phone system, which is designed primarily for voice and data. Its long-haul links have very high capacity -- increasingly based on optical fiber -- but the system is built primarily around the narrowband requirements of the telephone, plus other technologies (fax, computer modems) that can be made compatible with the characteristics of the ordinary phone. Twisted copper pair wiring remains the foundation of the local system.

A key characteristic is that this is a switched network. Each user has an address (the phone number) and the system is designed to route a call originating from any point on the network through a sequence of switches to reach the specific number being called. Most cable television systems, on the other hand, are distribution networks intended primarily to deliver programs from a central point to subscribers.

To many, Alexander Graham Bell and his colleagues seemed hopelessly visionary when in the 1870s and '80s they were describing telephone systems that would extend through cities much as the network of gas pipes did then, or when Bell predicted that businessmen would use the telephone to speak with "their agents a hundred miles away" as conveniently as they called their servants via their familiar household speaking tubes.

Mr. Bell and his successors were perhaps too modest in their projections. Consider some of the characteristics of the present-day telephone system:

- It is ubiquitous, extending virtually everywhere in the industrialized world and building rapidly elsewhere.
- Service is relatively inexpensive.
- It is a genuinely public network.
- The switched network configuration permits any two points in the system to be connected directly and virtually instantaneously.
- The system is growing rapidly in capability with advances in fax, data communication, and other technologies described above.

The phone system is an increasingly flexible resource. The switched telephone network has grown far beyond its "twisted copper pair" image. The phone companies are major users of optical fiber as well as high-capacity copper cable, they pioneered satellite communication, and they remain among the heaviest users of microwave systems. While we generally think of phone company services as narrowband, as noted above, these carriers commonly offer higher-capacity channels such as T1, which can transmit 1.544 megabits of information per second -- enough for many video applications. (see comparison charts, page 79)

Figure 1--The Public Switched Telephone Network

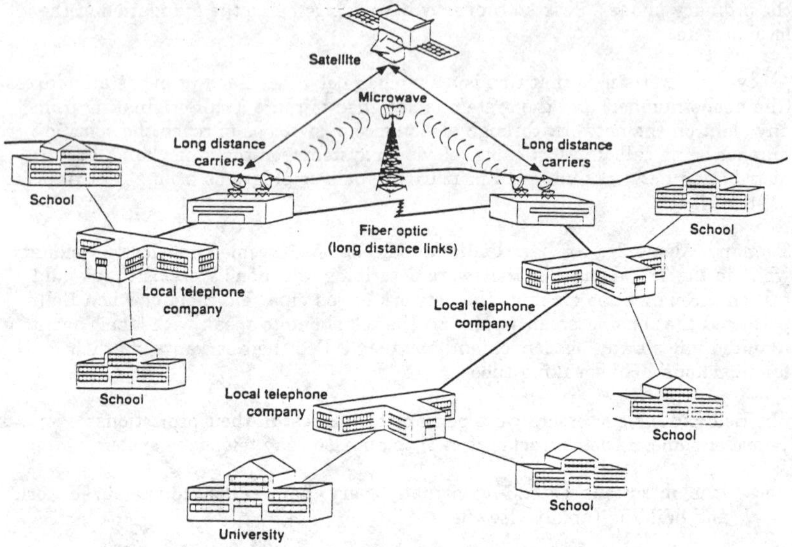

The public switched telephone network uses many technologies to connect subscribers near and far. Although used primarily for voice services today, in the future the public telephone network may become more a public information network, capable of carrying conversations, computer communications, and video programming.
SOURCE: Office of Technology Assessment, 1989.

At this writing the phone system of the United States consists of 22 Bell operating companies, several major independent telephone companies such as GTE, about 1400 smaller independent companies, and as many as 500 long distance companies.

The system is undergoing great changes, with more companies offering more services under a relaxed regulatory scheme, resulting in unprecedented ferment and innovation. The traditional rivalry between the telephone and cable TV industries is becoming a wary search for mutual benefit. America's future telecommunication system will be based on an integrated approach to voice, video, and data, with much more interaction by the user. Today's most fundamental trends are:

- The move toward wireless telephones and cellular systems. It is often predicted that the telephone system of the future will appear wireless to the user, with high-capacity cable trunks providing the infrastructure between wireless phones and terminals.

- The move to digital technology. This marriage of telecommunication and computing has several effects:

    a. It makes telecommunication systems much more versatile and flexible. Modern voicemail systems, for example, are possible because of digital switching and recording.

    b. It makes telecommunication systems more efficient, with resulting cost savings.

Case in Point: ISDN

Telecommunication users will be hearing much more about the Integrated Services Digital Network (ISDN), which is a practical application of the fact that to a digital transmission system, anything that can be sent is just a stream of off-on bits. In ISDN systems a variety of services can be sent through a single channel simultaneously, using a sort of mix-and-match coding that permits voice, data, etc., to be sorted out at the receiving end.

There are different sorts of ISDN interface, with varying capacities. Broadband ISDN (B-ISDN) is for users who need to handle large quantities of data, voice, and video simultaneously. Basic narrowband ISDN combines voice and relatively low-speed data. Primary narrowband ISDN can combine voice, data, and video at a bandwidth equivalent to a T1 channel. As might be expected, B-ISDN involves much more complexity in routing the various information streams to their intended destinations. As in many other areas of digital technology, however, distinctions and difficulties tend to blur as equipment evolves at an ever-increasing pace.

High Capacity (Broadband) Networks

Although the telephone system uses all the high-capacity transmission technologies, most people think of it as a narrowband service because of its historic emphasis on voice and compatible services, which are relatively undemanding consumers of bandwidth.

In this section we review the transmission technologies generally considered broadband. That is, they can carry a lot of information and often are associated with such voracious consumers of bandwidth as video.

In a rough order of capacity, they are microwave, coaxial cable, communication satellites, and optical fiber.

Microwave. Terrestrial microwave is a workhorse for relatively short-range wireless communication. Its distinguishing characteristic is that send and receive locations must be in line of sight. In the days before satellites and optical fiber (and not uncommonly today), transcontinental telephone and broadcasting networks marched across the continent via microwave repeater stations, mountaintop-to-mountaintop. Within urban areas microwave systems relay signals of all kinds point-to-point, located on convenient buildings or hills. The amount of bandwidth available varies from system-to-system, and depending on the application may be referred to customarily in megahertz or megabits. A common phone company microwave system has a bandwidth of 45 Mbps. Known as a DS-3 system, it can carry 672 phone lines or 28 T1 circuits. A local FM station relaying its programming from a downtown studio to its mountaintop transmitter may use a single-channel microwave system of 150 KHz. Suffice it to say here that microwave systems can be designed to meet widely varying requirements, digital or analog, and voice, video, or data.

ITFS. While the typical microwave system is highly directional (point-to-point), some varieties are intended to reach many locations (point-to-multipoint). During the 1960s such a microwave allocation was made to American education for the distribution of instructional television programming. In federal jargon it's known as the Instructional Television Fixed Service (ITFS), and a given educational licensee may use as many as four "conventional" six MHz channels. ITFS systems operate in the frequency band around 2.5 GHz (Gigahertz, or billion cycles per second), not far from UHF (ultrahigh frequency)[2] television stations.

---

[2] The sixty-eight channels available for broadcasting in the United States and Canada are divided into two groups -- very high frequency (VHF) channels [2-13] and ultrahigh frequency (UHF) channels [14-69].

Figure 2--Microwave Communication System

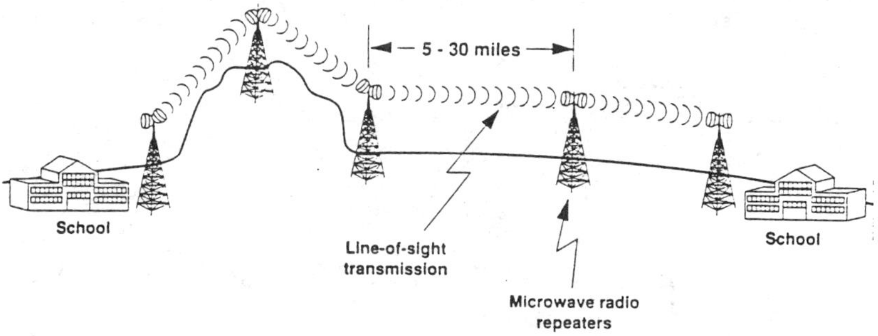

SOURCE: Office of Technology Assessment, 1989.

MMDS. The technology of ITFS is used also by the so-called wireless cable systems which offer television to home subscribers. This variation is known as Multichannel Multipoint Distribution Service (MMDS). Some MMDS systems in fact operate on the channels reserved for ITFS, through arrangements with local educational agencies.

With the advent of compressed video (described above) it is possible to fit multiple channels of video into the bandwidth previously required by one. As technology advances, that multiple keeps going up; at this writing it's possible to fit four to six channels into each "basic" channel.

Coaxial Cable. The technology used to send 30-to-50 channels of television into most American households is coaxial cable. The meaning of its name is clear if you examine a cross-section: a central conductor of copper approximately as thick as a pencil, a donut of insulating material, then another ring of conductor, and finally an insulating cover. This design enables the cable to handle much more bandwidth than ordinary twisted-pair copper wire, thus making multichannel cable television feasible. The capacity of any transmission system is gradually diminished as the signal travels over distance, and so systems are designed with amplifiers that boost the strength of the signals periodically. As is the case with all transmission media, the workable bandwidth available in coaxial cable systems is partly a function of the distance between amplifiers.

Figure 3--Cable Television Distribution System

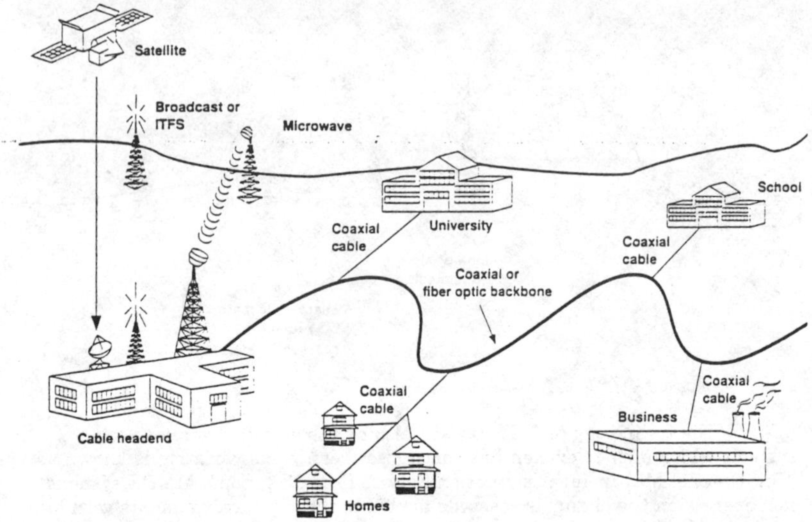

Programming from many sources can be redistributed through a cable television distribution system. Schools can receive educational programming through the local cable company and some systems can also be used for two-way communication between schools.
SOURCE: Office of Technology Assessment, 1989.

Incidentally, some people assume that coaxial cable is essentially a one-way medium, since most of us can't send signals back upstream from our television sets. In fact, this characteristic is simply a result of the fact that most cable companies (until recently, at least) have perceived themselves to be in the video distribution business, and thus have had no need for amplifiers that work in both directions. The limitation, then, is the amplifier and not the cable.

Communication Satellites. In the mid-1940s Arthur C. Clarke wrote an article that appeared in the journal *Wireless World*. It was called "Extraterrestrial Relays: Can Rocket Stations Give Worldwide Radio Coverage?" He described an orbit, 22,300 miles over the equator, where an object -- a "man-made moon" -- would appear fixed over a point on the earth's surface, neither rising nor setting. From such a position the object could "see" more than a third of the earth. If one could put a relay mechanism of some kind in that orbit, it would make possible instantaneous communication between virtually any two points over a third of the earth. If one could put such an extraterrestrial relay over each of the world's three great oceans, telecommunication could be virtually live, real-time, from nearly anyplace to anyplace on the planet. Furthermore, Clarke pointed out that during World War II the Germans had made great strides in rocket propulsion. With continuing advances in rocket technology such an orbit, he believed, soon would be achievable.

When he wrote his article, Arthur Clarke did not believe that his vision of communication satellites would be realized within his lifetime. But he hadn't counted on the invention of the transistor and the dawn of the microelectronics age, just a couple of years later. At this writing Arthur Clarke is alive and well, and satellites ring the earth precisely in the orbital positions he prescribed.

The communication satellite is a relay station in space. The pioneers in the field were microwave engineers. Accustomed to relays from mountaintops, they adjusted their calculations to design systems with a "mountain" 22,300 miles high, beyond our protective atmosphere in the vastness of space, with electric power provided by solar cells and batteries.

Like other broadband transmission technologies, a satellite can handle voice, video, or data. Satellites are now the prime carriers of broadcast and cable networks, and they are used increasingly for teleconferencing, delivery of course material, and other specialized purposes. While they are used in many telephone and data systems (much of the international traffic goes via Intelsat, the international satellite system), they introduce an annoyance: while their signals travel at the speed of light, the round trip of nearly 45,000 miles takes almost a quarter-second -- enough to disrupt the rhythm of normal conversation and an eternity to a computer's processor.

Satellites are designed with multiple channels of transmission. Within a satellite the fundamental relay device for a channel is the transponder. In many present-day satellites a transponder is equated with a video channel; for services demanding less bandwidth a transponder may be subdivided as necessary. With the advent of compression techniques, however, it is becoming possible for a transponder to handle multiple video channels simultaneously, thus dramatically reducing the cost per channel. In the past, a typical satellite had a dozen transponders, each with a bandwidth of 36 MHz, and a television channel took a full transponder. With today's compression technology, each transponder might handle four to eight channels of television, and even higher compression ratios have been announced.

Satellites also have ingeniously designed antennas, so that their transmissions may be focused on a given continent, country, or even a time zone or metropolitan region. Furthermore, focusing on a smaller footprint (as the coverage area is called) has the effect of increasing the power of the signal in that area, just as a flashlight's reflector increases the amount of light within a smaller area.

The familiar dish antennas that receive satellite transmissions collect energy radiated from the satellite, focus it on a central point, and deliver it to its destination. This antenna is also called an earth station or, not quite correctly, a downlink. Its diameter depends on the amount of energy that must be collected, and thus a signal of higher power can be handled by a smaller antenna. An earth station designed only to receive signals is of course much less expensive than one which also transmits (an uplink), and an earth station receiving simple analog television (like the typical backyard dish) is less expensive than the equipment necessary to handle compressed digital signals.

Figure 4--Satellite Communication System

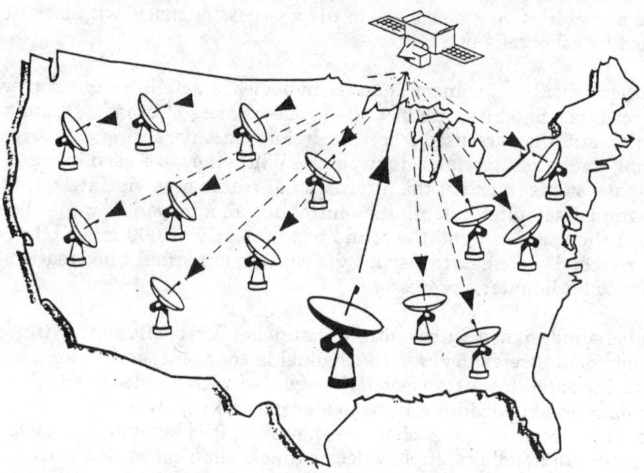

Satellites can deliver educational programming and courses to schools across the country. Video programming and text materials are broadcast from a central origination site (uplink) to any school with a satellite receiver (downlink). SOURCE: Office of Technology Assessment, 1989.

Satellite users find themselves in discussions of C-band and Ku-band satellites. These terms refer to the frequencies used: C-band satellites operate at lower frequencies than Ku-band spacecraft, 4/6 GHz vs. 11/14 GHz (a gigahertz is a billion wave cycles per second). These designations are also related to the services that carriers may offer with a given satellite.

Satellite systems have these principal characteristics:

- o Within the footprint of the satellite they can be received virtually anywhere. It's simply a matter of installing an earth station. Thus, these systems are very flexible.

- o For practical purposes, within the footprint of the satellite any transmission goes the same distance: 22,300 miles up and 22,300 miles down. Thus, charges are based on the amount of time and satellite capacity used in a transmission, and not on the distance between terrestrial points.

It should be acknowledged that satellites have a wide range of applications other than communication, including navigation, environmental and weather observation, military surveillance, etc.

Optical Fiber. If there is a glamour technology in telecommunication today, optical fiber is it. In addition to its relative novelty, there are some impressive reasons why:

- o Optical fiber offers enormous bandwidth, and succeeding generations of fiber get better and better. At this writing the highest-capacity fiber for commercial use has a bandwidth of 3.4 Gbps (gigabits per second), and most operate at 565 Mbps.

- o This bandwidth is in a very small package, making it especially attractive in areas where existing conduit is becoming overcrowded.

- o As the industry learns how to make ever more pure strands of fiber, fewer repeaters are needed to maintain the strength and reliability of the signal.

- o Since fiber systems use light rather than electricity, they are not subject to the electrical interference that plagues other systems.

- o The quality of the transmission in a fiber system is extremely high.

We hear that cable companies and the telephone industry are both moving rapidly to install fiber in their own plants. Will we have fiber to the home, thus making possible services undreamed of today? Maybe, but not soon. Here's why:

- o Although the cost of fiber is going down rapidly, and soon it may be cheaper to install fiber than copper, there is a huge standing investment in twisted copper phone lines and coaxial cable TV lines. Furthermore, not all the potential of those existing systems has been tapped.

- o Optical fiber systems transmit pulses of light, which must be converted to electronic signals before they can be used by your home television set or telephone. While fiber itself is becoming cheaper, there is a substantial cost in making the conversion from optical signals to electronic signals. At present it makes sense to make that conversion not in each home, but in the neighborhood (often referred to as "fiber to the curb".)

While fiber may not reach most homes for several years, it is increasingly common in institutions like hospitals, universities, and office complexes, because of its capacity, high quality, resistance to electrical interference, physical size, and decreasing cost.

It is now being used extensively in systems that handle huge quantities of phone, video, and data traffic, such as the trunk lines that carry great streams of information from city to city. Its capacity, quality, reliability, and decreasing demand for repeaters makes it the choice for transoceanic cable systems.

Its capacity and other characteristics, together with the costs of major installations and a more congenial regulatory environment, have invited partnerships and condominium arrangements in the development of fiber systems. Joint ventures between government and commercial carriers, or between phone companies and cable TV companies (normally arch rivals) are beginning to occur.

As costs come down and the demand for telecommunication goes up throughout our society, fiber is no longer only an urban or trunk-line phenomenon. Fiber systems are beginning to provide links for rural areas as well, and they can offer capabilities that most rural areas (indeed, most mid-sized cities) would have found infeasible only a few years ago.

Switches and Switching -- Making That Connection in the Public Network

No discussion of telecommunication/information technologies is complete without a brief discussion of the role of switches in a network. Understanding this component is particularly important to rural communities which seek to deploy new telemedicine technologies using the public switched telephone network.

Placing a call with the public network not only requires an input device (e.g., a telephone) and a means of transmitting the signal (e.g., twisted copper pair), but it also requires a means of routing the message through the network to its destination. This routing is accomplished with devices termed switches. One remembers perhaps the pictures of switchboard operators manually directing (switching) calls. Today, state-of-the-art digital switches are used by almost all the long-distance carriers. These switches, which are actually specialized computers, can connect more than 300,000 calls per hour. At many local exchange offices, however, electromechanical or electronic analog switches, earlier "generations" of switches, are still used.[3]

Because the public network contains several generations of equipment, problems can occur when compressed video signals need to be transmitted, as in telemedicine consultations. That is, transmitting the signals requires not only a high capacity channel (e.g., T1), but it also requires a digital switch to handle the transmission at the local telephone exchange. Therefore, when an institution or community is considering technology deployment, it should recognize that their carrier may have to install a new switch, as well as a new telecommunications line. This may have significant cost implications for the carrier.

Deciding on the Transmission System

Institutional Arrangements. When deciding on distance learning or telemedicine technology, institutions must consider not only the type of technology to purchase, but also how they will obtain transmission services. The choice of technology may actually be less important than the institutional arrangements used to obtain the services. Five common arrangements to explore are[4]:

- Dedicated networks - The institution installs, owns, and operates a specialized private network (this arrangement is common in education).
- Shared government networks - The institution shares capacity with a "private" state or local government network. Some states, however, prohibit a non-governmental entity, such as a private hospital, from using their network.

---

[3] Many independent rural telephone companies have been able to "leap-frog" to the new digital technology; i.e., they have gone directly from mechanical switches to digital switches. Many of their Bell counterparts are operating with electronic analog switches -- switches more advanced than the electromechanical, but not as advanced as the digital.

[4] This section is adapted from Parker and Hudson (1992, Chapter 3.) For examples in education see Parker and Hudson (1992); for examples in health care see Schmidt and Smith (in press).

- o Leased capacity from telephone carriers - The institution leases network capacity from the telephone carrier. Leasing network capacity is common for video and data services. Leasing may be the only way some telephone carriers offer access to fiber optic facilities.

- o Leased capacity from specialized carriers - The institution leases transmission capacity from a specialized carrier (e.g., a satellite corporation, a private commercial microwave or fiber network) for a monthly charge.

- o On-demand, "dial-up" networks - Under this arrangement, the institution is able to "dial-up" two or more circuits (e.g., 56 Kbps data circuits) as needed from a telephone carrier. This avoids institutions having to lease an entire line, when only occasional access is needed. Dial-up demand is often used with compressed video technology.

Cost Issues--The "last mile" barrier. Institutions in rural areas frequently face an issue termed the "last mile"[5] barrier. When rural institutions (e.g., hospitals) have begun to deploy these new technologies, some have discovered that the public network telephone lines to their facilities do not have sufficient bandwidth to carry the signals they need to send or receive. Thus, new line must be laid and the costs of its installation covered. Moreover, and as important, a new tariff (or rate) for the new line and service must be developed[6].

This new tariff may be extremely high. General telephone costs are low because the costs are spread over a large number of people. However, when a new line is provided and one facility is the major or sole user of the new high-capacity line, that facility may have to absorb the full costs of transmission services. For example, in the MEDNET project described in the next section, two hospitals to which land-based T1 lines were extended had to lease the lines around the clock, even though they used them only a small percentage of the time. The fixed monthly line charges for the T1 lines averaged $6,050 which, over a 12 month period, almost equaled the one-time equipment start-up costs at each hospital of $80,000.

A Note About Relative Costs. Among high-capacity systems -- microwave, coaxial cable, satellites, and optical fiber -- there are inevitable questions about relative cost. The core fact is that there are no enduring rules of thumb in these decisions: fiber is not always less expensive than satellite, or vice-versa; installing a

---

[5] The "last mile" is a term used in describing the laying of fiber optic cable. It to used to connote the distance from the major backbone of the carrier to the peripheral site. In actuality, the "last mile" may be a mile or, in some cases such as west Texas, it may be hundreds of miles.

[6] Local exchange carriers must file with the public utility commission for each different rate or tariff they offer to different customer groups (.e.g, business, residential, or university) and for different services (e.g., voice, data, video).

microwave system is a good solution in certain circumstances, but it may not be cost-effective if a fiber link with available capacity already exists. One must begin by comparing the requirements of the program with the characteristics of the available transmission systems.

To an increasing extent, the telecommunication industries face less regulation and costs are market-driven. Systems with excess capacity, or systems facing increased competition, may be prepared to offer incentives.

In review, key questions to be asked when making decisions concerning transmission systems, are:

About the program:
- How many sites are involved?
- Where are they?
- What is to be transmitted between/among them?
- How often and over what period?

About the transmission systems:
- What systems exist or are planned (by the local carrier, by the government, by other institutions)?
- To what extent will they meet the requirements of this program and other potential programs?
- What are their relative costs?
- Must tariffs be negotiated?
- Is a new system, built with this program as a sole major user, a realistic option? What would it cost?

Individual situations invite different solutions. Consider two systems, both of which focus on two-way interactive video: When the State of Oregon decided to proceed with its ED-NET system, it contracted with GTE for satellite service. The State of North Dakota, however, chose an optical fiber system which is also linked to a satellite-based rural hospital network. Both states believe they made the best, most cost-effective choice. Both may be right.

THE TECHNOLOGIES APPLIED TO RURAL HEALTH CARE[7]

This section will examine programs in which telecommunication technology is applied to rural health care. It is by no means a compendium of such projects, but rather a series of working illustrations intended to demonstrate situations in which these technologies have been applied effectively.

It should be emphasized that there is no cookie-cutter approach for applying technologies to problems. There are variables of cost, feasibility of technologies in given situations, information to be sent and to whom, etc. The important thing is to get the job done well, and often there is more than one way to do that. That is one of the lessons in the material below.

Projects Emphasizing Telephone-related Technologies: Phone, Fax, Slow Scan Video, Audiographics

Overcoming the Isolation of Rural Clinicians: The Maine Rural Health Center Clinician Support Network

Problem Addressed: Provide to rural areas a strong physician support system, such as those cultivated by medical schools and enjoyed by those in urban areas.

Technology Applied: Fax, speakerphone.

Program Summary: Maine, a largely rural state with mountainous terrain and harsh winters, has 28 community health centers serving more than 140 remote communities. The ability to maintain quality health care is diminished by the difficulty of persuading primary care clinicians to maintain practices in isolated areas, and health centers are hard pressed to overcome that isolation.

The Maine Rural Health Center Clinicians Support Network was created in October 1991 by the Maine Ambulatory Care Coalition (the state's primary care association), in association with the 28 member centers, the Maine-Dartmouth Family Practice Residency, and the Eastern Maine Medical Center Family Practice Residency. It was funded by a grant under the Rural Health Outreach Program of the federal Office of Rural Health Policy.

---

[7] Contact names for the following projects are provided in the CONTACTS FOR FURTHER INFORMATION section at the end of the document.

Key activities of the network include providing consultations among the 70 clinicians, and providing programs of continuing education (both formal credit courses and informal symposiums by teleconference). The telephone teleconferences have proven to be an effective vehicle for linking together the clinicians (whether they are at the hospital or the health centers), residency programs, and the presenters. Clinicians have found teleconferencing to be preferable to video-conferencing because it enables them to participate no matter where they are.

The fax system is used to support the consultation function by transmitting such diagnostic material as hospital EKGs. (For more applications of fax technology, see also the next entry, "More on Fax: Improving Medical Communication.")

Computer modems and Grateful Med Software (see the later entry) are now being provided to all the centers, along with training in their use. This will provide the clinicians at the health centers with another link to essential outside resources.

More on Fax: Improving Medical Communication in Hawaii

Problem Addressed: Improving medical communication between and within hospitals; making it possible for small hospitals to share resources of larger hospitals.

Technology Applied: Fax.

Program Summary: Hospital fax networks have been initiated in several areas, typically for administrative purposes. Analysis of a network established among hospital emergency departments in Hawaii in the 1980s showed that it had great promise for a wide range of applications, including:

Between Health Care Institutions
- Patient transfers
- Telephone patient consultation
- Instant medical records transfer
- Instant ECG interpretation
- Distribution of information from a central source
- Multicenter research links
- Central data collection and organization
- Instant retrieval of medical literature

Within Health Care Institutions
- Sending inpatient medication orders to pharmacy
- Sending lab and radiology reports to patient floors
- Sending supply requests to central supply

The establishment of fax capability in hospitals' emergency departments was advocated because they often serve as the hub for interhospital communication.

Although some of the above fax applications are being assumed by computer applications, fax technology continues to play an important role because of its simplicity and because it can use existing phone lines. Since the above study took place, new applications include using it to obtain signed medical consent in emergencies. One of the investigators in the fax study is now testing the feasibility of teleradiology using a personal computer.

Improving Diagnostic Capability in Rural Communities: Teleradiology and the Nevada Rural Health Project

Problem Addressed: Providing 24-hour access to radiologists for rural hospitals in Nevada (also see additional notes following the Nevada summary below).

Technology Applied: Computer-based image archiving and transmission system.

Program Summary: The Teleradiology Network of the Nevada Rural Hospital Project was launched in March 1990 with hospitals in eight rural communities -- Fallon, Lovelock, Winnemucca, Battle Mountain, Ely, Tonopah, Hawthorne, and Yerington, in conjunction with Medical Video Innovation. Hospitals in an additional three communities -- Elko, Boulder City, and Caliente -- are now part of the project. When the project began, three radiologists provided initial interpretations based on transmitted images, followed by formal written interpretation after receipt of the original films overnight.

In the original system, x-rays and CT films were placed on a camera light box table and viewed by a camera. The camera capture station digitized the film for transmission over the telephone line or for archiving. These digitized images were then transmitted from the rural hospital to a receive computer at the radiologist's station, monitored 24 hours a day. Sending and receiving physicians could view the same image simultaneously.

While this will remain the procedure for x-rays, in 1993 new equipment is being installed for use with CT and ultrasound equipment. In hospitals with CT or ultrasound equipment, a digitizing board is being added to the computer which is connected to the CT or ultrasound equipment. This will eliminate the need to take a picture of the developed film; rather the digitizing board will directly digitize the video signals from the CT or ultrasound equipment and immediately transmit them.

The hospitals within the NRHP have enjoyed a reduction in costs for patients and hospitals by reducing the number of patient transfers to larger, distant hospitals.

These data have been tracked by the NRHP office. Moreover, the community individuals are aware of the teleradiology systems, enhancing their overall view of available medical care. Last, the increased professional support for physicians has improved the ability of these rural communities to retain their physicians.

Comparable Projects. The Nevada project is not an isolated instance. Projects involving slow-scan or computer-to-computer transmission of diagnostic images have been reported from numerous other rural areas. Among them are western Nebraska, where a teleradiology program was established to spread scarce resources, ease staffing problems, and encourage physician recruiting by rural communities. Others include a program to provide the service of a radiologist to the remote community of Challis, Idaho, by Magic Valley Radiology Associates, P.A. and Sun Valley's Moritz Community Hospital; and that of Northwestern Radiological Associates, which provides services to two small hospitals and three offices in the Seattle area.

It should be noted that there is an ongoing issue of judgment concerning whether the quality of the transmitted image is high enough to warrant its use for final diagnosis. Such systems are commonly reported as comparable to a "wet" reading diagnosis, with final readings made from the original film. Image quality continues to improve, however, and it may be anticipated that an increasing number of radiologists will feel comfortable in using it as time goes on.

Continuing Education in Remote Areas: The Sioux Lookout Project in Northwestern Ontario

Problem Addressed: Provide continuing education to a remote area of northwestern Ontario, including CME programs, medical rounds, nursing rounds, in-service education, health professions student education, and patient education.

Technology Applied: Audio-teleconferencing and slow-scan video.

Program Summary: The Sioux Lookout Zone health care system provides preventive and curative health care to approximately 10,000 native people, over 80 percent of whom live in 27 villages scattered over 100,000 square miles. The zone hospital in Sioux Lookout is staffed with fourteen family physicians plus rotating pediatric and family practice residents from the University of Toronto. Specialty consultants visit the zone, but none live there.

There are fourteen nursing stations staffed by two-to-four nurse practitioners providing primary care under the supervision of the zone hospital. The other villages are served by health aides who are members of the local community and who are visited twice a month by a nurse located in the region.

Since 1978, the Sioux Lookout Zone Hospital has used teleconferencing to provide ongoing educational opportunities for nursing and medical staff. Nurses based at the nursing stations use teleconferencing to take turns presenting cases. Physicians also use teleconferencing to present cases, aided by consultants (e.g., in cardiology, dermatology, and radiology) in Toronto. Teleconferencing is also used for patient education and for medical and nursing student education.

From 1978 to 1990 the hospital used a slow scan network between four of the nursing stations and the zone hospital for diagnosis and consultations and transmitting x-rays, EKGs, charts, and video images of patients. However, new modes of transportation and communication have replaced the network. Airstrips have been established in all nursing station communities and patients are flown out daily if needed. EKGs are now transmitted using fax technology.

Sioux Lookout found that with a fairly rapid turnover of staff at the nursing stations, meeting the training needs to keep the system operational was difficult.

Audio-Conferencing with Existing Phone Lines: The South Dakota Medical Information Exchange for Training Physicians, Nurses, and Other Health Care Professionals

Problem Addressed: The need to provide education and updated information for diagnostic purposes.

Technology Applied: Audio-conferencing.

Program Summary: The University of South Dakota School of Medicine uses the South Dakota Medical Exchange (SDMIX) for continuing medical education across the entire state. There are over 30 rural teaching sites in addition to the major teaching campuses in Rapid City, Vermillion, Sioux Falls, and Yankton. Educational programs are available to all towns/cities in South Dakota, as well as being available nationally.

The educational programs are mostly clinically oriented and are one hour in length. Program format includes a forty-five minute lecture, supplemented with written materials and slides and/or video, followed by a 15-minute "live" interactive question and answer discussion. Program materials are mailed to each participating site two weeks prior to the date of the program.

More on the Use of Telephone-Related Technologies to Assist Health Care in Remote areas: The Experience of Memorial University of Newfoundland

The Memorial University of Newfoundland is a pioneer in the application of many telecommunication technologies for projects both domestic and international. While recognizing (indeed, helping to demonstrate) the efficacy of advanced video applications and new satellite technology, it was concluded in the late 1970s that many of the most important tasks could be accomplished with audio and related technologies, and that multipoint television would not be economically feasible in the Province of Newfoundland for the foreseeable future.

Accordingly, for more than a decade the university has been developing a province-wide system that is based on telephone conferencing, slow scan television, audiographics, and electroencephalograph and electrocardiograph transmission equipment. For the past year the Telemedicine Centre has been evaluating T1 land-based compressed video technology in health and education applications.

In planning its projects the Telemedicine Centre has applied these guidelines, which would be equally pertinent to many others:

- Use the simplest and least expensive technology that will meet needs.
- Develop a flexible system.
- Involve users (participants, audience, clients) from the beginning of the project.
- Seek the support of administrative personnel in hospitals, clinics, and other agencies.
- Plan carefully for the coordination of the system at all levels.
- Develop a consortium of users within and outside the health field.
- Plan for continuity of service beyond the demonstration project.
- Include evaluation.

Projects Emphasizing Computer Communication

Medical Information to Rural Practitioners: The GaIN Model of the Mercer University School of Medicine, Macon, Georgia

Problem Addressed: Deliver clinical medical library information to medical practitioners, medical students, and hospital personnel in Georgia.

Technology Applied: Microcomputer communication.

Program Summary: Established in 1983, the Georgia Interactive Network for Medical Information (GaIN) provides a 24-hour computer-to-computer link among rural Georgia medical practitioners, Georgia hospitals, and the Mercer University School of Medicine in Macon.

The project responds to the rapid growth -- and decreasing shelf life -- of medical information. Two reports of the Association of American Medical Colleges emphasized the need for increasing the ready availability of information and the parallel requirement for professionals to acquire information retrieval skills.

The mandate of the Mercer University School of Medicine (MUSM) is to help meet Georgia's need for physicians in rural and medically underserved areas of the state. The school thus provides services intended to address problems of professional isolation and lack of information services.

The GaIN system, which links remote microcomputers with a central computer at the university, involves three components:

- physician practice sites and remote clinical teaching facilities;
- hospitals;
- the GaIN Center at MUSM.

Through GaIN, participants may communicate by electronic mail and conferencing, receive advice from colleagues listed in a consultants' register, review educational opportunities on a CME bulletin board, and access biomedical literature through an online catalog and the GaIN MEDLINE. Bulletin boards, which provide current alert services and news services, are tailored to needs of specialized groups. Using electronic mail, physicians may use a librarian's services via their hospital libraries. GaIN can also be used as a gateway to a regional or national computer system, where additional information resides.

Physician Information Online Statewide: the University of Nebraska Medical Center

Problem Addressed: Provide timely information and communication services for health professionals throughout the Midwest.

Technology Applied: Computer Communication.

Program Summary: Synapse Health Resources Online assists in the provision of quality health care -- regardless of location -- by providing timely access to information and communication resources to health professionals. It is a service of the University of Nebraska Medical Center and University Hospital. The health professional, via personal computer, modem and phone line, can access the following:

- o Statewide electronic mail (over 6000 addresses),
- o medical, nursing, allied health, and pharmacy journal abstract databases,
- o online medical library card catalog and online library ordering,
- o the Nebraska Medicaid eligibility system,
- o the Nebraska professional licensure database,
- o multi-specialty bulletin boards,
- o continuing education case simulations (credit eligible),
- o drug interaction databases and drug information services,
- o online patient education materials (in Spanish and English),
- o Internet resources (list-serv, mail, FTP),
- o decision support and diagnostic aid databases,
- o Nebraska Peer-Reviewed Quality Guidelines,
- o AMA's practice parameters,
- o patient information (pre-reservation, discharge summaries, radiology, and lab results, etc.),
- o drug pricing and therapeutic equivalent database,
- o the University's bookstore online ordering system, and
- o various physician office management activities.

The network consists of over 600 health professionals in over 175 sites in seven states throughout the Midwest.

The University of Nebraska Medical Center (UNMC) also uses satellite and land-line based interactive audio/video for education and continuing education of health professionals in rural regions of the state (see state profiles). UNMC also provides telecardiology services to remote areas.

Physician Information Online Statewide: Oregon Health Sciences University

Problem Addressed: Provide information and communication services for practicing physicians.

Technology Applied: Computer Communication.

Program Summary: A service comparable to that of the University of Nebraska Medical Center is provided by Oregon Health Sciences University (OHSU). The Oregon system is ORHION (Oregon Health Information Online); it is a joint service of OHSU's Biomedical Information Communication Center and US HealthLink, a vendor of medical information services. ORHION is available via personal computer and modem 24 hours a day, seven days a week.

Among the services are:

- OHSU Medline, a five year, 1300 journal subset of the National Library of Medicine's Medline database,
- Access to 320 key medical journals via EMPIRES, Excerpta Medica Physicians Information Retrieval and Education Service,
- Photocopy service and document delivery via fax of mail,
- OHSU library catalog,
- OHSU bookstore service, online ordering and discounted prices,
- Electronic mail,
- Electronic bulletin boards on several topics,
- Comtex Medical News Service,
- Electronic clipping service for topics of the subscriber's choice,
- Clinical information including Medicom Drug Interaction Service, diagnostic support, and patient simulation modules (with CME credit available),
- Full-text reports including the Morbidity and Mortality Weekly Report from CDC Atlanta; the Communicable Disease Summary from the Oregon Health Division's Office of Epidemiology and Health Statistics; and summaries of clinically significant information learned during trials sponsored by NIH.

Extending the Services of the National Library of Medicine: Grateful Med and Loansome Doc

Problem Addressed: Provide access to the databases of the National Library of Medicine (NLM) to individuals in areas without access to a medical library. Provide a means to obtain full-text documents of citations retrieved through Grateful Med.

Technology Applied: Computer communication with the Grateful Med software package.

Program Summary: The MEDLARS family of databases maintained by the National Library of Medicine has long provided support to health professionals. In 1986 NLM introduced Grateful Med, a user-friendly, inexpensive software package that allows an individual, using a personal computer, to search NLM's MEDLARS databases.

In 1992 the Library added the Loansome Doc feature to the Grateful Med software. Loansome Doc enables individuals to order full-text articles from the references they retrieve in their Grateful Med search. The Loansome Doc feature is made available by a medical library in an individual's region with which an individual establishes an agreement for the service.

Virtual Medical Center and Healthnet

Problem Addressed: Isolation of rural health professionals.

Technology Applied: Computer, modem, and telecommunications software.

Program Summary: To decrease the isolation of rural health professionals, two Area Health Education Centers (AHEC), in collaboration with State Offices of Rural Health (SORH), have created and maintain electronic bulletin boards (EBBs) specifically for rural health professionals. The electronic bulletin boards -- "Virtual Medical Center" in Montana and "Healthnet" in Washington state -- serve as electronic information and education resources for rural health professionals. The bulletin boards include message areas where rural health professionals can leave private or public messages. Consulting networks and continuing education courses with x-rays and photographs will be available through the Virtual Medical Center. In-state access to these EBBs is available on a 1-800 number. Out-of-state health professionals can also sign-on to the EBBs, but are responsible for their long distance charges.

81-951 O - 94 - 8

Projects Using Broadband Communication Systems or Combinations of Technologies

Providing Specialty Consultation and Continuing Medical Education to Rural Patients and Physicians: The Medical College of Georgia Telemedicine Center

Problem Addressed: Expand the consultative services in all specialties offered at a teaching hospital to include patients in such facilities as rural hospitals, prisons, and community health centers. Provide continuing medical education credit to rural physicians for the time they spend in the interactive consultation with specialists.

Technology Applied: Video, personal computers, fax, medical telemetry via a land-based T1 link.

Program Summary: Through equipment currently based in the emergency room at the Medical College of Georgia (MCG) hospital, the MCG specialist and a physician in a rural hospital can examine a patient together. Technology includes remotely/locally controlled cameras enabling specialists to manipulate camera angles and zoom for detailed patient examination or viewing x-rays on a view box; a microcamera and series of adapters that capture the images from any scope at the remote site; and an electronic stethoscope. Other technologies allow real-time transmission of EKGs with freeze frame annotation and storage of patient images as slides. The system also includes personal computer applications for notes, patient records, and journal references. The network is about to begin a first phase expansion to 25 sites throughout the state.

To date, telemedicine has removed the need for transport of over 80% of patients seen over the network. MCG notes that retention of the patient in the community is improving continuity of care, bringing more timely care, and allowing patients to remain with their families during what is often a stressful time. Comparison of rural to urban daily patient bed costs suggests that retaining the patient at the local facility generally costs the health care system less.

Continuing Education for Rural Hospital Staffs: Oregon Health Sciences University and Northeast Oregon Area Health Education Center

Problem Addressed: Continuing education for health professionals in hospitals in rural northeastern Oregon, provided from Oregon Health Sciences University in Portland.

Technology Applied: Satellite-based one-way video with two-way audio.

Program Summary: The eight hospitals in the Northeast Oregon AHEC (NEOAHEC) have been fitted with receive-only satellite dishes plus audio talk-back in order to receive continuing education programs from Oregon Health Sciences University in Portland. Initial courses were directed to physicians, but courses in nursing and allied health are now also provided.

The program uses the Oregon ED-NET system, which has three networks:

- Network 1 (used in this program) consists of one-way video delivered by satellite, with two-way audio. When fully developed, Network 1 will have about 600 locations throughout the state for receive-only video and two-way audio.

- Network 2 consists of satellite-based interactive compressed video. There are 40 two-way interactive video sites statewide, and a transmission originating from any of them can also be made available via Network 1. Thus, in addition to the "live" interactive sites on Network 2, other sites may receive video and participate by audio.

- Network 3, known as Compass, is a dial-up computer communication network and is terrestrial rather than satellite-based. It provides a variety of information services, including user-friendly access to local, national, and international databases, government and academic libraries, computer conferencing, and electronic mail. Very remote rural sites have local access numbers to the Compass network. It is being used extensively in nursing education and a project is being initiated among nursing executives in the region for sharing details on educational opportunities jointly available among their institutions.

Baccalaureate Programs for Nurses: the Approaches of Hawaii, New Mexico, and Oregon

Problem Addressed: Make it possible for practicing nurses located in rural areas to complete baccalaureate or masters programs in their home communities.

Technology Applied: Video, audio, ancillary technologies. Various approaches are illustrated by the three cases.

Program Summaries. Hawaii, New Mexico, and Oregon are addressing essentially the same problem: how to make baccalaureate or masters' programs in nursing available to practicing nurses in rural areas. All use telecommunication. From the standpoint of the students the approaches are similar, but distinctly different technical systems are employed. The essential lesson is that different systems, chosen as best in their respective situations, can provide similar service.

The three systems are as follows:

The University of New Mexico. One-way video via satellite plus two-way audio by telephone is used to transmit five courses per year to about 30 sites, which are located in rural hospitals or community colleges. Courses are offered live, with live phone connections to the students wherever they may be. Video transmissions are also captured locally on VCRs.

Two clinical courses are not involved in the broadcast schedule. Lower division courses may be taken from community colleges. Completion of the program normally takes about two years of continuous enrollment beyond the lower-division requirements.

The University of Hawaii at Manoa. The University of Hawaii at Manoa offers a Master of Science in Nursing outreach program. The instructional approach is similar to New Mexico's, but the technical system involves a combination of point-to-point microwave and ITFS, all part of the Hawaii Interactive Television System (HITS). The HITS system reaches the islands of Oahu, Kauai, Maui, and Hawaii, with origination possible from the islands of Hawaii (the University of Hawaii at Hilo), Maui (Maui Community College), Kauai (Kauai Community College), and Oahu (the University of Hawaii at Manoa, Kapiolani Community College, Leeward Community College, Honolulu Community College, and the State Department of Education).

Oregon Health Sciences University. In Oregon both the basic nursing baccalaureate curriculum and the RN/BS completion program are offered to selected sites throughout the state. The technology employed is two-way compressed "live" video via Oregon ED-NET's Network 2 and computer conferencing for class assignments via Network 3. (As noted above, ED-NET Network 1 is a one-way video with audio return satellite network; Network 2 is a two-way video, two-way audio network using digital video compression; and Network 3 -- Compass -- is a low-speed computer communications network. Networks 1 and 2 are satellite-based, while Network 3 is terrestrial-based.)

The telecommunication system is seen as integral to the long-term development of nursing programs in Oregon. The state's nursing programs are being merged, with OHSU as the lead institution. Providing the program to local communities via telecommunication is central to the planning process.

Note: Nursing programs require clinical practice. In these programs clinical components are arranged through local hospitals where appropriate supervision is available, or faculty members travel to assure that clinical work is completed satisfactorily.

Training Health Professionals in Rural Areas: Interactive Video in North Dakota

Problem Addressed: Provide people in rural areas an opportunity to receive training in health professions, and respond to the shortage of health professionals in the state.

Technology Applied: Interactive video via an optical fiber network and satellite.

Program Summary: Bachelor of science degree programs in nursing, social work and medical technology are offered from the University of North Dakota, using two-way interactive video and audio.

North Dakota has an optical fiber network linking the state's public colleges and universities and the state capitol. This Interactive Video Network (IVN) is intended as the first step toward making broadband service available throughout the state. Fourteen classrooms equipped with optical fiber links currently comprise the network. The fiber system is now being complemented by (and linked to) a satellite system called MEDSTAR, which has receive-only dishes in 32 rural hospitals.

Statewide Continuing Education for Physicians, Nurses, Other Hospital Staff, and Patients: The Health Communications Network of the Medical University of South Carolina

Problem Addressed: Provide an ongoing program of continuing education to physician, nurses, allied health professionals, administrators, hospital support staff, and patients.

Technology Applied: Video transmitted via microwave; telephone.

Program Summary: The Health Communications Network of the Medical University of South Carolina is a full-color broadcast facility. The Medical University maintains a full-service production studio facility; State teaching hospitals in Greenville, Columbia, and Spartanburg maintain production origination capabilities. The network provides over 120 hours of continuing education programming each month, reaching an audience of 25,000 to 30,000 health care providers and consumers each year. Programming is broadcast to more than 75 on-site classrooms in South Carolina, linking more than 50 hospitals and state agencies.

In addition, the Network's microwave system is used to transmit two-way video/audio interactive undergraduate and graduate courses among the Medical University of South Carolina, the University of South Carolina School of Medicine, Clemson University, Spartanburg Regional Medical Center, Greenville Hospital System, and Richland Memorial Hospital. One-way video, two way audio teleconferencing facilities via satellite are also available.

Improving Rural Health Care in West Texas: Three Successful Telecommunications Demonstration Projects - MEDNET, KARENET and Tech Link

Problem Addressed: Improve rural health care and health professions education in West Texas and alleviate professional isolation.

Technology Applied: T1 compressed interactive video, satellite-delivered video, slow-scan video (static imaging), facsimile, computer network.

Program Summary: The MEDNET pilot program began in 1989 with a major federal grant. Activities initiated under MEDNET are now continuing under Texas Tech's HealthNet organization.

The four elements of the former MEDNET program are:

- Clinical consultations between generalists and specialists facilitated by T1 lines carrying two-way compressed video, audio, graphics, and data. Patients at two rural hospitals, Alpine and Ft. Stockton, can be "seen" at Health Sciences Center facilities in Lubbock, Odessa, or El Paso. In August 1993, the T1 link was extended from the hospital in Alpine to a small rural health clinic in Presidio, Texas on the Mexico-Texas border. With this link, physician assistants (PA) in Presidio can consult with physicians in Alpine. When the link is completed, the Presidio clinic will also be linked to Odessa and Lubbock allowing the PAs to consult with HSC's specialists.

- High-quality static imaging for transmission of X-rays. Other diagnostic material (e.g., text) is transmitted using personal computers.

- Continuing education - including grand rounds, case conferences, seminars, and workshops for physicians, nurses, and other health care professionals. One-way video via satellite, with two-way phone interaction is used to deliver CE at 46 hospitals.

- o Fax equipment. Originally installed in 19 sites to facilitate document transfer from the Health Sciences Center libraries, doctors quickly found that they could use the system effectively for fetal monitoring consultations. (This reduces the number of patients who would otherwise be automatically referred to specialized care centers.)

A report on the MEDNET program summarized its benefits as follows:

- o Made possible physician-to-physician and physician-to-physician assistant or nurse practitioner consultations without geographic limitations.
- o Kept patients in local care settings, increasing patient revenues at the home facility and reducing the expense of patient travel for both the patient and taxpayer.
- o Allowed rural health professionals to receive and participate in continuing education programs locally, at greatly reduced expense to the local hospital.
- o Decreased professional isolation.
- o Increased the availability of diagnostic resources.
- o Improved access to current medical literature.
- o Helped support and supervise health professions students in rural training sites.
- o Increased the confidence of rural patients in their local physicians and hospital and enhanced the rural hospital and community's ability to attract and keep primary care physicians and staff.

The Kellogg Affiliated Remote Environments Network (KARENET), Texas Tech's first health network, was funded under a grant from the W.K. Kellogg Foundation. KARENET used computers, with staff-developed software programs, to link sites in El Paso, Lubbock, and rural Morton. The computers provided access to a variety of services, including patient management protocols, on-line conferencing for medical consultations, access to an automated health care record system, continuing health professions education programs, and patient education programs targeted to community health needs.

Tech Link, a video conferencing network operating on a T1 line, was initiated in 1987 to connect the Texas Tech Health Science Center in Lubbock with its three rural academic health centers in El Paso, Amarillo, and Odessa. Tech Link is used to provide lectures to students at the four medical school campuses and is also used for administrative purposes (e.g., faculty and staff meetings).

After the potential of these projects was demonstrated, Texas Tech created HealthNet in 1992. HealthNet integrates these three demonstration projects and other rural health outreach projects into a comprehensive effort addressing West Texas' rural health needs.

Oregon's RODEO Net: Meeting the Needs of Mental Health Service Providers in Rural Areas

Problem Addressed: Advance the purpose of the Eastern Oregon Human Services Consortium to provide for the cooperative management of mental health programs, and to develop and operate specialized mental health services in as cost-effective a manner as possible.

Technology Applied: The three networks of Oregon ED-NET: one-way video with two-way audio; two-way interactive video and audio; and a dial-up computer network.

Program Summary: The goals of the RODEO Net Project are as follows:

- Improve patient care through increased access to and communication with necessary resources.

- Develop a well-trained and confident mental health workforce in remote communities by enriching ongoing training and staff development opportunities using telecommunication technologies.

- Determine if telecommunications is a cost-efficient and effective means of service delivery.

- Encourage policies that reflect the changing nature of service delivery in the use of telecommunications, particularly in the area of funding public mental health services.

Using interactive video telecommunications, RODEO Net provides services such as 24-hour crisis response for persons suffering extreme emotional or behavioral turmoil; mental health case consultation with physicians and other professionals; pre-admission services and pre-discharge interviews; and pre-commitment hearings.

The training function of RODEO Net includes one staff development certificate program for professionals and paraprofessionals working with children who have severe emotional disturbances; two staff development certificate programs in the planning stages; individual training sessions as requested by regional steering committees or sessions that take advantage of guest speakers or training programs at other sites; and a post-masters' program in psychiatric/mental health nursing from Oregon Health Sciences University for a small group of nurses at the Eastern Oregon Psychiatric Center.

Reducing the Isolation of Rural Practitioners: Mountaineer Doctor Television (MDTV)

Problem Addressed: Demonstrate the value of telemedicine consultations for reducing isolation of practitioners and enhancing access to specialist care in rural areas.

Technology Applied: Two-way compressed interactive video and audio via dedicated T1 terrestrial phone lines.

Program Summary: Based at West Virginia University Health Sciences Center, the Mountaineer Doctor Television project will link the Health Sciences Center (HCS) to four hospitals, providing for 24-hour video consultations and emergency assistance between rural physicians and the specialists at HSC.

The program will also include interactive continuing education for health professionals, as well as training for students of the health professions and residents who are doing rural clinicals. In addition, the system will be used for weekly grand rounds and to provide the nursing program to students in a rural community. The MDTV program began with its first continuing education program and its first telemedicine consultation to one hospital site in July 1993. Three additional hospitals will be added within a year.

Exploring the Potentials of the Internet for Community Hospitals: Pilot Connections in the Pacific Northwest

Problem Addressed: Explore the efficacy of providing health professionals in community hospitals, including rural community hospitals, with access to networking and health information resources via the Internet.

Technology Applied: Advanced computer communication.

Program Summary: Perhaps this project should be categorized with other projects emphasizing computer communication, but its scope suggests a home with these programs which use combinations of technology, including broadband systems. Based at the University of Washington, the project is coordinated by staff of the Regional Medical Library and the hospital librarians at the project sites. The project is assisted by NorthWestNet, the regional computing and communications network which manages the regional sub-unit of the Internet. The Pilot Connections program is conducted through the university's Regional Medical Library contract program with the National Library of Medicine.

The program's overall goal is to explore optimal technical, financial, and user models for extending network access to community hospitals. The program's objectives are:

- To assess the costs, benefits, and relative suitability to community hospitals associated with dedicated, multi-user network access vs. dial-up, single-user access.

- To observe the extent to which networked information resources and services -- made accessible by way of network connections -- are introduced to and used by hospital staff, and note the factors that seem to affect this in the various settings.

Seven community hospitals in five states are involved in the project. Three of the hospitals are connected to the Internet using 56 Kbps dedicated line connections for simultaneous multi-user access; four hospitals are connected using dial-up access.

Individuals at the seven sites are using their new access for:

- e-mail and electronic discussion groups,
- participating in continuing education programs offered online,
- communicating with a defined group of colleagues for such purposes as the business of a professional organization,
- checking the FDA Bulletin Board for information on the status of drugs,
- collaborating on reports and professional writings,
- quickly and inexpensively searching the databases and databanks of the National Library of Medicine,
- quickly obtaining the full-text of journal articles or book chapters with high resolution,
- transmitting datasets, such as abnormal chromosome laboratory results which are lengthy, complex, and difficult to transcribe accurately,
- checking late-breaking weather reports for emergency airlift pilots,
- searching the catalogs of libraries all over the world.

Testing of document image transfer hardware and software (Ariel) began in March of 1993. The equipment and software program allow the librarians to scan pages of books or journals and transmit these as files over the Internet. This is used for interlibrary loans in lieu of photocopying and mailing, or faxing, and is cheaper, faster, and provides a document of a higher quality. The participating community hospitals are:

Alaska Native Medical Center, Anchorage, Alaska
Kootenai Medical Center, Coeur d'Alene, Idaho
Kalispell Regional Medical Center, Kalispell, Montana
Shodair Children's Hospital, Helena, Montana
Merle West Medical Center, Klamath Falls, Oregon
Providence Hospital, Everett, Washington
St. Peter Hospital, Olympia, Washington

Statewide TeleHealth Projects

Many telemedicine initiatives have been singular projects based out of single entities, eg., universities - (MEDNET at Texas Tech University, MDTV at the University of West Virginia, the telemedicine project at the Medical College of Georgia). In some states however, the movement in telecommunications has been at the state level -- for health care, education, health professions education, or rural development.

GEORGIA: Georgia's "Distance Learning and Telemedicine Act," passed in 1992, allocates $50 million from telephone company over-earnings to finance state telecommunications projects in medicine and education. Specifically, the act directs the state Department of Administrative Services (DOAS) to develop, implement, administer, and manage a consolidated, integrated, statewide, shared-use distance learning, and telemedicine network. As the first step in doing so, the needs of the educational and medical communities are being defined. Based on this information, DOAS will make decisions about transmission technology alternatives. A Distance Learning and Telemedicine Board has been established to oversee and administer the fund.

IOWA: Three years ago Iowa legislators passed an act to create a statewide fiber optic network[8], the Iowa Communications Network (ICN). ICN was initially constructed to provide educational opportunities for Iowans from K-12 through the university level and also to provide access for state government and libraries. A large portion of the costs of network construction has been covered by issuing bonds. The educational use of the network is subsidized, providing particularly inexpensive educational rates.

Recently, it has been suggested that ICN be opened to health care providers as a means to enhance health care services in rural Iowa. A consortium of Iowa hospitals and universities has been pursuing a cooperative venture with the ICN to develop a statewide medical information network -- the "Iowa Medical Information Network." In July of 1993, the consortium demonstrated specific health applications on the network.

KANSAS: In Kansas, a state-wide telemedicine planning initiative was jump-started with a grant from the Kansas Health Foundation. The Foundation jointly funded the Kansas Hospital Association and the Kansas Department of Health and Environment to study possible applications of telemedicine in Kansas. The goal of the initiative is to develop materials to help educate individuals about telemedicine and to provide a structured approach for evaluating and implementing telemedicine applications in Kansas.

A public/private policy group comprised of the range of players -- government representatives, health care providers, insurers, educators, and interested others -- was established to guide the project. A four-volume report has been developed for communities to use to evaluate their telemedicine applications. This includes an overview of current telemedicine applications, an overview of policy issues, a community planning guide for telemedicine, and a source book of references.

NEBRASKA: In the late 1980's, the Nebraska Educational Telecommunications Commission recommended that its 25-year-old nine-transmitter microwave system, used to deliver educational television, be updated. Agreeing, the state legislature funded NEB*SAT -- a satellite and fiber optic system. The system's backbone is a transponder on the Spacenet III satellite. The system is capable of simultaneous broadcasting on three networks: a broadcast-quality TV channel for ETV and public radio, a second broadcast-quality channel for distance learning, and narrow-band channels for compressed video (16 one-way or 8 two-way

---

[8] The ICN is a synchronous optical network (SONET) with transmission speeds up to 2.4 gigabits per second. The 2.4Gbps network of Phase I will link Iowa's three regent universities and 15 community colleges in regional centers, the state capital, Iowa Public Television, and the Iowa Network Control Center at the Iowa National Guard Armory in Camp Dodge. The 84 links of Phase II, which will extend the links from the regional centers to the remaining counties and support 565Mbps transmission speeds, will tie in primary high schools and community college branch campuses. Phase III links will tie in most high schools on leased connections.

channels).

The system is available for use by all University of Nebraska campuses, state and private colleges, technical and community colleges, the state Department of Education and public radio. It is currently used to deliver nursing, medical technology, and other health science education classes. It is also used for academic administrative meetings and for continuing education programs.

NORTH DAKOTA: In North Dakota, telehealth telecommunication efforts initially focused on health professions training needs for individuals in rural communities. Under a grant from the Department of Agriculture, the University of North Dakota and North Dakota State University collaborated to establish the "Rural Health Distance Education Project" in 1989. The project offers entire health professions degree programs in 14 classrooms throughout the state using a two-way interactive video system - IVN (see project description, page 35).

OKLAHOMA: The Oklahoma Medical Information Network (OMIN) is a three-year pilot project funded by a restitution fund from the U.S. Department of Energy. (The fund was established by DOE to redress gas and oil overcharges between 1973 and 1981.) Under phase one, a teleradiology system is being established to link six rural medically-underserved sites with the University of Oklahoma Health Sciences Center. Under phase two, an information system for data retrieval via computer will be implemented, and under phase three, interactive video teleconsultations will be established.

PENNSYLVANIA: Pennsylvania Governor Robert Case announced plans in May of 1993 for the Pennsylvania Rural Health Communications Network (HealthNet). This network will be instituted in three prototype phases, the first to begin in October 1993. The network will connect understaffed and underequipped rural hospitals and community health centers with larger, better-equipped hospitals via two-way video/audio connections, teleradiology, and computer-to-computer conferencing.

SOUTH DAKOTA: South Dakota's "Rural Development Telecommunications Network" (RDTN) grew out of a telecommunications task force formed in 1990 by the late Governor Mickelson. The network was developed with funding from a variety of sources, including a Federal Energy Conservation grant and a Future Funds grant secured by the Governor's Office of Economic Development. The network came on-line in December of 1992, first hooking-up six educational institutions in the state. Education has priority for scheduling and the recent hook-up of three hospitals -- one rural facility and two urban tertiary care centers -- is for educational and administrative purposes. Discussions are being held to explore the use of the network for medical video consultations.

TELEHEALTH AND USER SUPPORT

Those involved in telemedicine and its close relation, distance learning, recognize that it is not enough to install the equipment, turn it on, and find people who want to use it. Support is required at several points. The purpose of this section is to point out common areas in which support is essential if programs are to succeed.

Is the System Ready? The world has all too many disgruntled souls who have tried technology and found it wanting. The dreaded line, heard often when we gather in professional conferences, is, "At our place we tried [fill in the technology] and it didn't work." Most commonly behind this complaint is either of two situations:

- o For any of several possible reasons the system became operational before it was fully installed and thoroughly tested. Its start-up glitches were revealed, its backers were embarrassed, and potential users, understandably enough, avoided it. The technology was blamed for the failure.

- o The early users of the system were not properly trained and supported. They floundered, the system seemed clumsy and reaction was poor. It was concluded that the technology didn't work.

Training of Users. At the very least it is necessary to acquaint users with the technology and the situations in which it will be used. The purpose of this training is not to burden them with technical detail, but to make users sufficiently familiar with the equipment that they can use it comfortably and recognize the opportunities and constraints that are built in.

For those taking part in a telephone conference, the problem is minimal: recognize the need for some protocol in managing the session, so that all can participate equitably so that votes can be taken or consensus recognized, etc.

For those responsible for presenting a multi-site two-way video course or consultation, the need for training is greater. It's not complicated, but it takes practice and attention.

Example: For those who wish to use the technology to provide medical consultation, thought must be given during the design phase to such issues as the location of the equipment in the health facility, the portability of equipment, operation and control of the equipment, and the elements of camera-patient-clinician interaction. Then, with adequate training and support, those who use the system can concentrate on the business of the moment, not distracted by the machinery of the system.

Training of Students. Health professions training programs that are preparing students for rural practice also share a responsibility for training students in the use of some of these technologies. At a minimum, students should be trained in the use of computers to search medical/health information databases and exposed to other electronic information and networking resources.

Ongoing Technical Support. Those in the health professions are well aware of the need for regular, competent maintenance and upgrading of hospital equipment. There is a similar requirement for telecommunication systems. While the equipment in the systems described above is relatively stable and hardy, regular maintenance is essential.

Furthermore, the technology is developing so rapidly that an important part of technical support consists of tracking change, recommending equipment updates when there are significant advances or when it becomes more economical to replace equipment than to maintain it.

Technical support at the operational level -- operating or monitoring equipment when a consultation or course session is in progress -- is also important in many systems and can be critical to the success of the program.

Technical support is an area which too often receives little attention, inevitably to the detriment of the program's success.

REGULATORY, LEGAL, AND QUALITY ASSURANCE ISSUES

This section provides a basic overview of some of the regulatory, legal, and quality assurance issues confronted by those implementing telecommunication systems. For more detailed discussions about these issues, please refer to the resource section of this publication.

Frequently, individuals in education and health care who are considering investing in telecommunications systems focus first on the technology and its capabilities. However, the regulations guiding telecommunications infrastructure and services will have a significant effect on how distance education and health care services will be made available to rural areas. A basic understanding of the players and issues is therefore important. As Ellen Wagner[9] has pointed out, it is critical for users of these systems to be aware of some of the complexity in order to insure their best interests are being served and that they are paying the right price for the services needed to serve the public. Moreover, such an understanding is critical if those in health care and education are to influence telecommunications policy decisions.

The education community has been involved to a greater degree and for a longer period of time in utilizing telecommunication technologies than has the health care community. Although in the early 1970s there were a few small telecommunication projects serving health care needs in rural areas, there was little activity in the area during most of the 1980s. It has only been within the last few years that a critical mass of health professionals and facilities has begun using these technologies. Thus, it is only recently that the need has arisen in the health care community to examine, as the educational community has done for the past decade, the legal, regulatory, reimbursement, and quality issues surrounding telecommunications utilization.

The Regulatory Players

Telecommunications regulatory authority and policy making are shared by a range of public sector players including: the *Federal Communications Commission (FCC)*, an independent federal agency responsible for coordinating the use of the airwaves and with oversight over broadcasting, cable, and telephone industries; the *National Telecommunications and Information Administration (NTIA)*, Department of Commerce, the executive agency responsible for coordinating executive branch telecommunications policy; *federal courts* which administer decisions affecting the industry (e.g., the Modification of Final Judgment that resulted in the breakup of the Bell System); *state public utility commissions*, responsible for regulating intrastate and local telephone service; and *state and local authorities*, responsible for regulating local cable franchises (U.S. Congress, OTA, 1989: 150).

---

[9]. Some of the information presented here was developed by Ellen D. Wagner while a visiting faculty member with the Western Cooperative for Educational Telecommunications. A more thorough examination of the regulatory environment can be found in Dr. Wagner's chapter, "Regulatory Issues in Distance Education," in B. Willis (Ed.) *Distance Education: Strategies and Tools*. Englewood Cliffs, NJ: Educational Technology Publications. It is scheduled to be published in January 1994.

Higher Education

Legal concerns surrounding tele-education involve a range of issues, including the implications of interstate telecommunications instruction and possible conflicts between states' rights to control education and the constitutional prohibition against their regulating interstate commerce. They also include issues relating to potential first amendment constraints, equal protection, restraint of trade, civil rights, and the determination of "physical presence" of an institution in a state (Chaloux, 1985 as noted in Reilly and Gulliver, 1992).

One of the first attempts to grapple with these issues in higher education was the Project ALLTEL (the Project on Assessing Long Distance Learning via Telecommunications - 1982-1984). Co-sponsored by the Council on Postsecondary Accreditation (COPA) and the State Higher Education Executive Officers Organization (SHEEO), Project ALLTEL specifically addressed issues of state authorization and voluntary accreditation relating to higher education delivered using telecommunications across state lines. The project also helped frame the legal, regulatory, and quality assurance context for telemediated education. As a result of Project ALLTEL, COPA and SHEEO issued a policy statement on "Accreditation and Authorization of Distance Learning Through Telecommunications in 1984."

A later effort in education, the 1990 invitational symposium on "Emerging Critical Issues in Distance Higher Education," also focused on quality assurance in distance education, as well as regulatory and accreditation issues. The symposium, convened by the Regent's College Institute for Distance Learning, the Annenberg/CPB Project, and the American Council on Education, noted the need to establish a research agenda that would inform policy development in distance learning.

The latest effort in this arena is a 1993 project that includes most of the players in these earlier efforts. The Western Interstate Commission for Higher Education's (WICHE) Western Cooperative for Educational Telecommunication is working with the educational policy makers of 15 western states to establish mutually compatible standards for telecommunicated interstate degree programs. A similar effort is under way in the Southeast headed by a regional higher education accrediting agency.

Although the higher education community has grappled with, and addressed, quality issues since the 1980s, it faced a significant challenge even as late as 1992. In 1992 legislation was introduced in the Congress that would have declared instruction delivered via telecommunications to be correspondence study. The rationale was that instruction provided via telecommunications technology was not of the same quality as that offered in a face-to-face situation. In higher education, such a decision would have dramatically affected students' eligibility for financial aid as well as the funding of telecommunication projects. The educational telecommunications community mobilized to inform key congressional staff about the scope of current activities in this arena and the potential impact of such legislation on students. The result was legislation that defined a broad scope of telecommunicated classes that were separated from the category of "correspondence courses."

Health Care

Many of the issues addressed by the educational community have counterparts in the health care arena, with specific health care twists. For example, the health care community is now beginning to address the following issues:

- Quality of health care delivered by telecommunications,
- Reimbursement of care delivered by telecommunications -- in particular video-to-video consultations[10],
- Licensure of health professionals who deliver telemediated care across state lines,
- Privacy issues in terms of patient information in clinical networks and clinical consultations, and
- Protocol development for participation in telemedical consultations.

Just as those involved in tele-education grappled with issues relating to the quality of telemediated coursework, the health care community is now confronting issues relating to the quality of telemediated consultations. And, as in education, decisions based on concerns about quality have dollar ramifications. Many public and private health care insurers are not yet willing to reimburse for telemediated care (i.e., remote diagnostics and consultations) because of concerns about quality, efficacy, safety, and costs. The Health Care Financing Administration (HCFA), which administers the Medicare and Medicaid programs, has given its regional offices authority to determine whether they will pay for telemedicine services. However, many of them are waiting for a stronger mandate from HCFA headquarters before they reimburse for services. Many private insurers who have historically followed HCFA's lead in reimbursement policy are likewise waiting.

[10] Telepathology and teleradiology, which involve the transmission of computerized data and images, are already covered by many insurers.

Rural health care facilities and professionals are also confronting regulatory and quality assurance/liability issues that relate to their ability to access health information services for health care delivery. For example, the Joint Committee on Accreditation of Healthcare Organizations (JCAHO) has revised its standards for 1994 to require hospitals to provide access to authoritative and up-to-date print and non-print information resources in a timely and efficient manner. For many small rural hospitals unable to maintain these sources in a print format, electronic access to information resources may be the only cost effective means by which they will be able to meet such standards. Similarly, rural clinicians' access to the latest clinical information also is increasingly important in terms of quality of care and related professional liability issues. Physicians are being held responsible for searching the current literature to seek, find, and apply the latest medical information when treating patients (Montana Task Force for Biomedical Information, 1993).

Several activities are now underway to address health care telecommunications issues. The federal Office of Rural Health Policy is convening an invitational workshop in November 1993 to identify and address the major barriers, including regulatory and policy barriers, inhibiting the diffusion of telemedicine to rural communities. In mid-1993, the Health Care Financing Administration contracted for a survey of the current uses of telecommunications technologies in expanding access to health care and an analysis of these uses as they relate to the development of Medicare coverage policy.

The Rural Electrification Administration is funding a major demonstration program to develop and expand the rural applications of telecommunications technology for distance learning and health care. The National Library of Medicine funds an outreach initiative to provide health professionals in rural areas with access to information services. More recently, as part of the High Performance Computing and Communications (HPCC) Initiative, NLM has solicited proposals to advance the medical applications of advanced computing and digital communications. Finally, telemedicine issues are being addressed by the American Telemedicine Association. ATA was founded in 1993 to promote professional, ethical, and equitable improvement in health care delivery through telecommunications technology.

Cost of Access

Another critical problem for those involved in providing education and health care in rural areas using telecommunication technologies is that of cost. Not only do rural areas need access to technologies that are comparable to those in urban areas, such access must be comparably affordable. The small populations and large distances of the rural regions are generally incompatible with the economies of scale that characterize many aspects of telecommunications. As a result, market forces rarely work to benefit rural areas. As the Congressional Office of Technology Assessment has pointed out, regulatory mandates and incentives are frequently necessary.

To understand some of the regulatory issues surrounding costs, the concept of tariffs must be understood. The United States Public Switched Telephone Network (PSTN) evolved as a monopoly. Consequently, telephone service providers do not operate the way most businesses do in a free-market system. The rates they can charge are controlled by a state public utility (or service) commission.[11] Thus, a carrier cannot simply decide what price to put on a service. Rather, it must file a price schedule, called a tariff or rate, with its regulatory commission. Once the regulatory commission approves the rate, the services are offered at those standard prices to any user.

Most tariffs in use today were designed primarily for voice and data transmission and may be inappropriate for the capacity required for video transmission (Koch, 1991). Thus, pricing policy -- especially for video services -- is still evolving as telephone companies gain more experience with video transmissions and processing technologies. Because no standardized price structure or tariffs exist for multi-channel video service, telephone companies are pricing services on a case-by-case basis.

Institutions considering installing new systems should investigate the pricing structure available from their carrier. They should be prepared to negotiate rates, which may entail waiting several months for the regulatory approval of a new rate. And they should be aware that because state public utilities set the tariffs. the rates for services will vary from state to state, as well as within states depending on the circumstances in the community.

As noted earlier, the Texas Tech MEDNET project had to lease a T1 line around the clock, even though they used it only a small amount of that time. This was because they were not successful in negotiating for on-demand access.

Players in education and health care are now recognizing, and beginning to address, needed regulatory reforms at both the federal and state level. Such reform includes providing incentives for telecommunication carriers to develop alternate pricing for educational and health care applications. For example, in a 1991 Congressional hearing chaired by New Mexico Senator Bingaman, several

[11] The tariffs and price structures for communication facilities set forth by PUCs are intended to allow telephone companies a fair rate of return on their capital investments.

witnesses called for national policy recommendations dealing with specific regulatory reforms to reduce the cost of common carrier telecommunications charges for educational purposes.

Several states have already instituted regulatory reform. In 1989, the Kansas Corporation Commission began to allow regulated telephone carriers, on a case-by-case basis, to implement reduced "Economic Development Rates" for services provided to certain types of entities, including educational organizations. Tennessee's Public Service Commission (PSC) developed two special educational tariffs. The first rate is for basic phone line service to elementary and secondary schools. The discounted rate is specifically for lines used for computer connections to information databases in classrooms and teachers' workrooms and for lines used by teachers to place outgoing calls to parents. This PSC also established a second educational tariff for high capacity private lines to educational institutions (i.e., T1 lines capable of transmitting interactive video signals). This second educational tariff is 50% less than the rates paid by other private line customers.

Copyright Issues: While these developments indicate enhanced access to telecommunications resources for educational groups (and the potential for similar access for rural health care), there are still many issues that need to be addressed. No one has solved the problems that arise with the United States' copyright system when intellectual material is "published" electronically and can be available on a network that is accessible to anyone with a computer, modem, and telephone line. There are some experimental projects, mostly in the library community, but no single solution exists (and may never). The ability to address this issue will affect how quickly such applications are available to the general public. This has particular significance for health professionals in rural areas where access to extensive print-based collections are limited.

Interoperability/System Compatibility: The interoperability (or compatibility) of different communication systems is another issue that must be addressed. Regulatory agencies, responsible for establishing rates, also set standards and protocols necessary to insure compatibility among communications systems. This allows different systems to communicate with each other, important in both education and health care. This is particularly important for rural communities. For example, Nebraska is served by 42 different telephone companies with different operating systems and technological bases. In order to be able to provide telemedicine services over these lines, interoperability must be assured.

Evaluation and Research

The effectiveness of the use of telecommunication technologies for secondary and post-secondary education is fairly well documented. Students studying at a distance tend to score about the same on tests as their counterparts in the face-to-face sessions of the same class. In many cases, students studying at a distance perform better than students in traditional classes probably for two reasons: (1) the off-site students are typically older, more motivated students than those studying on the campus, and (2) classes taught using technology frequently are designed more systematically to create a successful learning experience for the students.

For example, all the materials for the course are developed for specific learning goals and can take advantage of a variety of technologies. Those parts of the course content that require a verbal explanation (lecture) can be videotaped for students to view at the appropriate point in the course. This tape can last as long as it needs to and does not have to conform to a specific number of minutes of scheduled classroom time. Discussions can be scheduled on selected topics using computer conferencing or audioconferencing that might include a particular expert in the field. "Papers" can be written and revised and shared with groups of class members using electronic communication. Students can have access to the faculty member on a one-to-one basis through electronic mail, voice mail, or telephone calls.

There is far less evaluative information specifically on the effectiveness of distance learning for health professions education and continuing education. Although educators have been studying media-assisted learning for over 50 years, there are few studies on its utilization in the health professions, particularly with newer technologies.

There is also little evaluative material on the effectiveness of telemedicine as a means of providing care -- both in terms of clinical effectiveness and cost-effectiveness. This is in part because most telemedicine projects are recent endeavors. Moreover, the current emphasis in medicine on outcomes research, including quality, appropriateness, and cost-effectiveness of care, is a fairly new phenomenon. The Medical Treatment Effectiveness Program, the major federal effort to understand and address practice variations, was established in 1989.[12] Efforts in telemedicine to study issues of clinical effectiveness as well as cost-effectiveness are thus hampered by a lack of research and research models in the field overall.

---

[12] This research program is managed by the Federal Agency for Health Care Policy and Research, one of the eight agencies of the U.S. Public Health Service, DHHS.

Evaluation and research in health professions distance education and telemedicine are needed if these applications are to be successfully developed and effectively used in rural America. Rural communities need guidance before they invest scarce resources in expensive equipment that may not be adequate or appropriate for their needs. Federal agencies and decisionmakers need additional information to assure that new rural telemedicine projects are appropriate and effective. Reliable information about how well different technologies work for different purposes, the relative costs of those technologies, and the lessons that were learned by the pioneers in this field, could help others avoid the same mistakes and improve on the efforts of others.

CONCLUDING COMMENTS

Rural Networks and Superhighways

The telecommunications infrastructure is undergoing rapid growth and change. Information and telecommunication technologies are being developed and deployed at an ever increasing pace. The regulatory arena is in great flux as it attempts to adjust to the constantly changing environment. In this new information age the danger exists that telecommunications technologies and sources of information may be inequitably distributed, tilting toward overabundance in urban areas and scarcity in rural areas. Rural communities have an opportunity to help shape what they will have available to them. Health professionals knowledgeable about the options can help their rural communities make wise choices.

Rural Area Networks (RANS)

Rural communities differ in the telecommunications infrastructure currently available to them. Some rural communities, because of their size or location, may have ready access to a range of telecommunication channels and long distance carriers. However, many communities do not and, as the Congressional Office of Technology Assessment has noted, many rural communities may not be able to afford more than one modern high capacity telecommunications network.

The Congressional Office of Technology Assessment has recommended the creation of Rural Area Networks (RANS). In contrast to Local Area Networks (LANS), which are built around functional lines, RANs would be configured around the geographic boundaries and needs of an entire rural community. Aggregating the telecommunication needs of health providers, educational institutions, businesses, and local government, would enhance economies of scale and scope, as well as provide greater leverage in the marketplace for the community and its diverse sectors.

The development of a such a network is an option that rural communities may want to explore. New organizational arrangements as well as regulatory flexibility would be required for this strategy to work. Whether or not that option is feasible for a community, the planning for telecommunications infrastructure is critical. A troubling phenomenon seen in many rural communities is the lack of coordinated planning among different potential users (e.g., education, health care, and business). Telecommunication technologies are increasingly being deployed to meet individual sector needs, rather than being visualized and planned for as an

Figure 5--Rural Area Networks

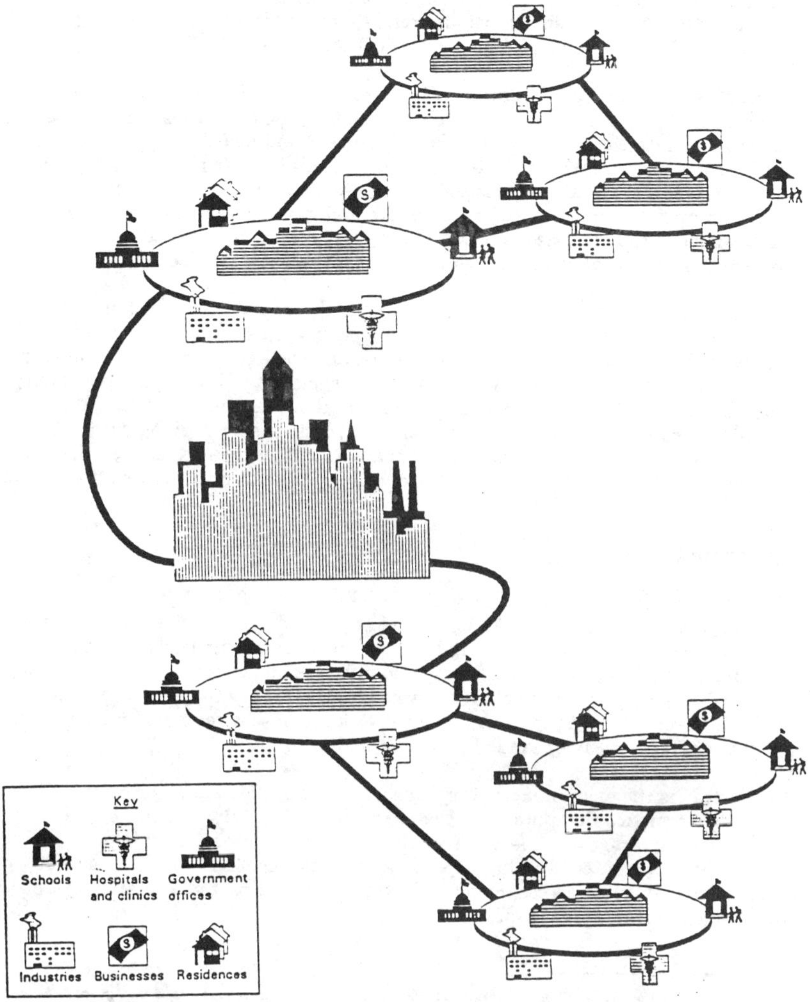

A Rural Area Network would be designed to foster the deployment of advanced technology to rural areas in an economically viable manner by pooling the communication needs of a community's many users--especially the businesses, educational institutions, health providers, and local government offices.
SOURCE: Office of Technology Assessment, 1991.

infrastructure element of the community (such as roads, or water or sewage plants). The result is that in some rural communities, different telecommunication systems serve different sectors, a situation that may not be the most cost-effective, viable situation for a community as a whole.[13]

The opportunity exists for rural health professionals, and others active in rural health, to play a critical role in not only enhancing the overall success of a health facility, but also the overall economic development and health of a community. To address the telecommunication infrastructure needs of their rural communities, health professionals can help foster needed new partnerships: between telecommunication experts and rural health and rural development experts, between rural communities and their state regulators, and between technical experts and the rural communities whose future is being decided.

For example, rural health providers can bridge the gap between regulators who rarely consider multifaceted economic development goals when making regulatory policy, and other health providers, educators, and local governments who often are not aware of what is at stake for them in the regulatory process. An opportunity now exists for educational, health care, and rural development individuals to influence important telecommunications policy decisions by working with regulatory agencies. Regulatory agencies are all public agencies and, as the education community has begun to learn, can be influenced by requests that serve the public good.

Superhighways

One reads more and more in the popular press about the new "electronic superhighway" -- particularly in its relation to a new world of video entertainment and interactive services. Receiving less attention, but particularly important to health care and education, is the proposed information superhighway -- the National Research and Education Network (NREN). As proposed, the NREN will be an interconnected gigabit computer network system for research and education -- in essence, a greatly expanded and enhanced Internet.

The NREN is the electronic networking component of the federal government's "High Performance Computer and Communications Initiative" (HPCC). The HPCC is an interagency federal research and development effort in high performance computers and high-speed communication. In FY 1993, over $800 million was budgeted across agencies for this initiative, part of a total budget of $5 billion for the next four years.

---

[13] Deaconess Medical Center in Billings recently launched an innovative demonstration telemedicine project in Eastern Montana that also addresses rural community development. For the first six months of the demonstration period, the network will be available at no cost for business and community service purposes.

The Administration has endorsed applying the technologies developed under the HPCC initiative to health care and education in two recent reports -- "A Vision of Change for America," a report that accompanied President Clinton's address to the Joint Session of the Congress, and a February 22, 1993 White House technology policy paper. Applications proposed include linking schools, hospitals, libraries, and other entities to the high-speed network; supporting technology to provide health care providers with access to relevant medical information and literature; and developing collaborative technology to allow providers in remote locations to provide real-time treatment of patients, etc.

Rural health providers can work to ensure that the proposed information superhighway -- the National Research and Education Network (NREN) -- does not bypass rural America. As can be seen in the Pacific Northwest Pilot Connections project, the NREN has the potential to enhance access for rural health providers to biomedical and other information databases -- access that can maintain and enhance the quality of care in rural health facilities and decrease the isolation of rural health professionals.

CONTACTS FOR FURTHER INFORMATION

PROJECTS

Maine Rural Health Center Physician Support Network
Bonnie Post, Executive Director
Maine Ambulatory Care Coalition
P.O. Box 390
Manchester, ME 04351
207-621-0677, FAX 207-621-0577

Hawaii - Inter-Hospital Faxing
Dr. Loren G. Yamamoto
Department of Pediatrics
John A. Burns School of Medicine
University of Hawaii
1319 Punahou Street
Honolulu, HI 96826
808-956-6525, FAX 808-949-4232

Nevada Teleradiology Activities
Nevada Rural Hospital Project
4600 Kietzker Lane, Suite A-108B
Reno, NV 89502
702-827-4770, FAX 702-827-0190

Sioux Lookout Project - Ontario Canada
Sioux Lookout Zone Hospital
Box 1500
Sioux Lookout
Ontario, Canada P8T 1C2
807-737-3030, FAX 807-737-3138

South Dakota Medical Information Exchange
Connie Kleinsasser
Network Program Coordinator, SDMIX
School of Medicine
University of South Dakota
2501 West 22nd Street
Sioux Falls, SD 57117-5046
605-339-6638, FAX 605-335-2869

Memorial University of Newfoundland
A.M. House, MD, FRCPC
Professor of Medicine
Associate Dean, Professional Affairs
Faculty of Medicine
Memorial University of Newfoundland
St. John's, Newfoundland, Canada, A1B 3V6
709-737-6645, FAX 709-737-7054

GaIN - Georgia Interactive Network for Medical Information
Jocelyn A. Rankin, Ph.D., Director
Medical School Library
Mercer University
1550 College Street
Macon, GA 31207
912-752-2519, FAX 912-752-2051

SYNAPSE - University of Nebraska Medical Center
Robin K. Meter, SYNAPSE Coordinator
Department of Computing Services and Telecommunications
University of Nebraska Medical Center
600 South 42nd Street
Omaha, NE 68198-5030
402-559-5759, FAX 402-559-5579

ORHION - Oregon Health Information Online
Steve Teich, Coordinator for Outreach Programs
Biomedical Information Communication Center
Oregon Health Science University
P.O. Box 573
Portland, OR 97207
503-494-3444, FAX 503-494-5241

Grateful Med Software and Loansome Doc Services
National Library of Medicine
8600 Rockville Pike
Bethesda, MD 20894
301-496-6193 or 800-638-8480

To Order Grateful Med Software:
National Technical Information Service
5285 Port Royal Road
Springfield, VA 22161-0001
703-487-4650, FAX 703-321-8547

To obtain information on libraries in one's area that provide Loansome Doc service, contact your Regional Library of the National Network of Libraries of Medicine (NN/LM) at 1-800-338-7657.

Virtual Medical Center (VMC)
Robert Flaherty, M.D.
Montana Area Health Education Center
333 Culbertson Hall
Montana State University
Bozeman, MT 59717
406-994-5738, FAX 406-994-6993

Healthnet - Washington Rural Health Electronic Bulletin Board
Lorraine Edwards
Office of Community and Rural Health
Department of Health
P.O. Box 47834
Olympia, WA 98504-7834
206-753-5942, FAX 206-753-9100

Medical College of Georgia Telemedicine Project
Jay H. Sanders, M.D.
Director of Telemedicine
Telemedicine Center
Medical College of Georgia
Augusta, GA 30912-1655
706-721-6616, FAX 706-721-7270

Oregon ED-NET
Raymond Lewis, Ph.D., Director
Christy Leonhardt, Director of Marketing
7140 Southwest Macadam Ave., Suite 260
Portland, OR 97219
503-293-1992, FAX 503-293-1989

Continuing Education Services on Oregon ED-NET
Sandy Ryman, Executive Director
Northeast Oregon Area Health Education Center
Eastern Oregon State College
1410 L Avenue
LaGrande, OR 97850
503-962-3801, FAX 503-962-3416

Telecommunicated Baccalaureate Nursing Degree Programs
Joanne Itano, Ph.D., R.N., O.C.N.
School of Nursing
University of Hawaii at Monoa
2528 The Mall
Honolulu, HI 96822
808-587-3312, FAX 808-587-3360

Dianna Shomaker, Ph.D., R.N.
College of Nursing
Nursing/Pharmacy Building
University of New Mexico
Albuquerque, NM 87131-1061
505-277-5725, FAX 505-277-3970

Mary McFarland, Ed.D., R.N.
Oregon Health Sciences University
School of Nursing
3181 Southwest Sam Jackson Park Road
Portland, OR 97201
503-494-3658, FAX 503-494-4350

Marcia Shoup Short, M.S., R.N., Associate Director
School of Nursing at East Oregon State College
Oregon Health Sciences University
Hunt Hall, 304-B
LaGrande, OR 97850
503-962-3645, FAX 503-962-3737

North Dakota - Rural Health Distance Education Project

Jack M. Geller, Ph.D., Project Coordinator
The Center for Rural Health
University of North Dakota
School of Medicine
501 Columbia Road
Grand Forks, ND 58203
701-777-3848, FAX 701-777-2389

Judith A. Euller, Ed.D., R.N.
Director, Distance Education in Nursing
University of North Dakota
College of Nursing
P.O. Box 8195
Grand Forks, ND 58202-8195
701-777-4508, FAX 701-777-4096

South Carolina's Health Communications Network

Jerry Mallard, Director
Medical University of South Carolina
Division of Television Services
171 Ashley Avenue
Charleston, SC 29425-2920
803-792-4435, FAX 803-792-4987

Texas HealthNet (includes the former MEDNET program)

William T. McCaughan, Executive Director
Steve J. Cotton, Director of Marketing and Program Development
Texas Tech University Health Sciences Center
HealthNet
HSC 1C162
3601 4th Street
Lubbock, TX 79430
806-743-2640, FAX 806-743-2233

Mountaineer Doctor Television (MDTV)

Robert D'Alessandri, M.D.,
Vice President for Health Sciences
Dean, School of Medicine
James Brick, M.D., Medical Director, MDTV
WVU Health Sciences Center
P.O. Box 9000
Morgantown, WV 26506-9000
304-293-4511, FAX 304-293-4973

RODEO NET

Douglas C. Overlock, Executive Director
Catherine Britain, Project Manager
RODEO NET
Eastern Oregon Human Services Consortium
P.O. Box 2905
La Grande, OR 97850
503-963-9393, FAX 503-963-2189

Pilot Connections in the Pacific Northwest

Sherrilynne Fuller, Ph.D., Director, Health Sciences Library and Information Center
Director, National Network of Libraries of Medicine (NN/LM), Pacific Northwest Region
Neil Rambo, MLibr, Associate Director
National Network of Libraries of Medicine, Pacific Northwest Region
University of Washington, SB-55
Seattle, WA 98195
206-543-8262, FAX 206-543-2469

STATE ACTIVITIES

Joe Werner
Manager of Tariffs
Tennessee Public Service Commission
460 James Robertson Parkway
Nashville, TN 37243-0505
615-741-2791, FAX 615-741-2336

Richard Morrissey
Office of Local and Rural Health Systems
Kansas Department of Health and Environment
Landon State Office Building
900 S.W. Jackson
Topeka, KS 66612-1290
913-296-1200, FAX 913-296-1231

James P. Larson, Executive Director
Rural Development Telecommunications (RDT) Network
500 East Capitol Avenue
Pierre, S.D. 57501-5070
605-773-3333; FAX 605-773-6581

Iowa Communications Network (ICN)
Department of General Services
Division of Communications
Hoover State Office Building
Level A
Des Moines, IA 50319
515-281-3336; FAX 515-242-5974

James Logan, M.D.
Oklahoma Medical Information Network (OMIN)
Oklahoma University Health Sciences Center
Provost's Office
P.O. Box 26901
Library Building, Room 221
Oklahoma City, OK 73190
405 271-2332; FAX 405-271-3150

James Anderson, Director
Strategic Network Development
Department of Administrative Services
Telecommunications Division
200 Piedmont Avenue, Suite 1402
Atlanta, GA 30334
404-651-6393; 404-656-7074

Reba Ann Benschoter, Ph.D.
Director, Biomedical Communications
NEB*SAT
University of Nebraska Medical Center
Box 985170
600 South 42nd Street
Omaho, NE 68198-5170
402-559-7100, FAX 402-559-7103

James Reid, Director
Eastern Montana Telemedicine Project
P.O. Box 37000
Billings, MT 59107
406-657-4870; FAX 406-657-4875

Leslie Best, Coordinator
HealthNet
Pennsylvania Department of Health/Governor's Office of Telecommunications
Bureau of Primacy Care Resources & Systems Development
P.O. Box 90
Harrisburg, PA 17108
717-772-5298; FAX 717-783-3794

The Medical College of Georgia, Robert B. Greenblatt, M.D. Library maintains a telemedicine database. Information about the database and service charges can be obtained by calling the library at 706-721-3667.

To obtain copies of the four volume telemedicine report jointly prepared by the Kansas Department of Health and Environment and the Kansas Hospital Association contact:

Office of Local and Rural Health Systems
Kansas Department of Health and Environment
Landon State Office Building
900 S.W. Jackson, Room 1051
Topeka, Kansas 66612-1290
913-296-1200
FAX 913-296-1231

American Telemedicine Association
P.O. Box 200195
Austin, Texas 78720
800-899-1101

REFERENCES AND ADDITIONAL READINGS

Byers, Steven. 1991. *Using Distance Education in Human Resource Development - A Report of a Western States Mental Health Conference*. Boulder, Colorado: Western Interstate Commission for Higher Education.
[WICHE, P.O. Drawer P, Boulder, CO 80301-97524]

Chaloux, Bruce. 1985. *Assessing Long Distance Learning Via Telecommunications - Project ALLTEL: A Summary Report*. Washington, D.C.: Council on Postsecondary Accreditation and the State Higher Education Executive Officers Association.

Faculty Development Subcommittee of the Western Cooperative for Educational Telecommunications. 1991. *Faculty Resource Guide to Distance Education*. Boulder, Colorado: Western Cooperative for Educational Telecommunications (WICHE).
[WICHE, P.O. Drawer P, Boulder, CO 80301-97524]

Gammon, Deede. 1991. *Telemedicine in Northern Norway*. TF R 27/91. Teledirektoratets forskningsavdeling.

Gilcher, Kay, and Sally Johnstone. 1988. *A Critical Review of the Use of Audiographic Conferencing Systems by Selected Educational Institutions*. College Park, Maryland: International University Consortium, University of Maryland.

Indiana Department of Commerce. 1991. *Lifelines to Rural Indiana - The Role of Telecommunications in Rural Economic Development*. Indianapolis, Indiana: Indiana Economic Development Council, Inc. [317-631-0871]

Invitational Symposium on Emerging Critical Issues in Distance Education. 1990. *The Proceedings of the Invitational Symposium on Emerging Critical Issues in Distance Higher Education*. Sponsored by Regents College - the University of the State of New York, The Annenberg/CPB Project and American Council on Education. Available from the Institute for Distance Learning, Regents College, Albany, New York. [518-474-3703]

Koch, Susan. 1991. *Telecommunications and Economic Development in the Great Lakes Region*. Bloomington, Indiana: Institute for Development Strategies.

Krebs, Arlene. 1991. *The USDLA Funding Sourcebook for Distance Learning and Educational Technology*. Tustin, California: Technological Horizons in Education Journal.

81-951 O - 94 - 9

Lenn, Marjorie Peace, Ed. 1991. *Distance Learning and Accreditation.* Washington, DC: Council on Postsecondary Accreditation.

Levine, Toby Kleban. 1992. *Going The Distance: A Handbook for Developing Distance Degree Programs Using Television Courses and Telecommunications Technologies.* Washington, DC: Corporation for Public Broadcasting and Public Broadcasting Service.

Little, Arthur D., Inc. 1992. *"Telecommunications: Can It Help Solve America's Health Care Problems?"* Cambridge, Massachusetts: Arthur D. Little, Inc.

Markwood, Richard, and Sally Johnstone. 1992. *The New Pathways to a Degree Project Evaluation: First Year Report of the Annenberg/CPB Project.* Boulder, Colorado: Western Cooperative for Educational Telecommunications (WICHE).
[WICHE, P.O. Drawer P, Boulder, CO 80301-97524]

Milio, Nancy. (1991) Information Technology and Community Health -- Invitation to Innovation. *Journal of Professional Nursing* 7(3), 146.

MITRE Corporation. 1990. *MITRE Conference on the Expanding Role of Telecommunications in Health Care -- Telehealth 2000.* McLean, Virginia: The MITRE Corporation.
[The MITRE Corporation, Civil Systems Division
7525 Colshire Drive, McLean, Virginia 22102-3481]

Montana Task Force For Biomedical Information. 1993. *Report to the Governor: Montana Task Force [for] Biomedical Information.* Helena, Montana: The Task Force. Contract No.: N01-LM-1-3506. Available from Montana State Library, Helena, MT 59620.

National Aeronautics and Space Administration (NASA). 1992. *International Telemedicine/Disaster Medicine Conference: Papers and Presentations (December 9-11, 1991) NP-207.*

Norwegian Telecom Research. 1992. *Applied Telemedicine.* Tromsoe, Norway: Troms Trykk A/S.

Nymo, Birger J. and Bjorn Engum. 1990. *Telemedicine to improve the quality, availability and effectiveness of the health service in rural regions.* A paper presented at "Seminar on the Regional Impact of Advanced Telecommunication Services", Kiruna, 19-21 June 1990.

Office of Science and Technology Policy, Federal Coordinating Council for Science, Engineering, and Technology, Committee on Physical, Mathematical, and Engineering Sciences. (1993) *Grand Challenges 1993: High Performance Computing and Communications - The FY 1993 U.S. Research and development Program.*

[Committee on Physical, Mathematical and Engineering Sciences, c/o National Science Foundation, 1800 G St., N.W., Washington, DC 20550]

Parker, Edwin B. and Heather Hudson, with Don A. Dillman, Sharon Strover, and Frederick Williams. 1992. *Electronic Byways: State Policies for Rural Development Through Telecommunications*. Boulder, Colorado: Westview Press, Inc.

Reilly, Kevin and Kate Gulliver. 1992. Interstate authorization of distance higher education via telecommunications: The developing national consensus in policy and practice. *The American Journal of Distance Education (6)*2, 3-16.

Schmidt, Ronald E. and Gregory L. Smith. (in press) *Telemedicine: Assessing the Kansas Environment. Volume 1: The Role of Telemedicine in Health Care Delivery; Volume II: Telemedicine Policy Issues; Volume III: Community Telemedicine Planning Guide; Volume IV: Telemedicine Source Book*. Topeka, Kansas: Kansas Department of Health and Environment and the Kansas Hospital Association.

Texas Tech University Health Sciences Center. (1993) *Texas Tech MEDNET: A Bridge for Rural Health Care - Demonstration Project Summary Report.*

U.S. Congress, Office of Technology Assessment. 1989. *Linking for Learning - A New Course for Education*. Washington, DC: Government Printing Office.

[GPO Stock Number: 052-003-01170-1 ($9.00)]

U.S. Congress, Office of Technology Assessment (OTA). 1990. *Critical Connections: Communication for the Future*. OTA-CIT-407. Washington, DC: U.S. Government Printing Office.

[GPO Stock Number: 052-003-01143-3 ($17.00)]

U.S. Congress, Office of Technology Assessment. 1990. *Health Care in Rural America*, OTA-H-434. Washington, DC: U.S. Government Printing Office.

[GPO Stock Number: 052-003-01205-7 ($22.00)]

U.S. Congress, Office of Technology Assessment (OTA). 1991. *Rural America at the Crossroads: Networking for the Future*. OTA-TCT-471. Washington, DC: U.S. Government Printing Office.

[GPO Stock Number: 052-003-01228-6 ($9.50)]

The federal reports listed above are for sale by:
Superintendent of Documents
U.S. Government Printing Office
Washington, DC 20402-9325
202-783-3238

U.S. Department of Commerce. 1991. *The NTIA Infrastructure Report - Telecommunications in the Age of Information*, NTIA Special Publication 91-26.
[NTIS order #: PB 92 10-248-2. ($25)]
For sale by:
National Technical Information Service
5285 Port Royal Road
Springfield, VA 22161-0001
703-487-4650

Willis, S. 1989. *Distance Education Through Telecommunications: A Directory of NUCEA Institutions Utilizing Telecommunications in Distance Education*. Washington, DC: National University Continuing Education Association.

GLOSSARY OF TELECOMMUNICATIONS TERMS

Amplifier - electronic devices, spaced at intervals throughout a cable television system, used to boost the strength of the cable signal as it passes from the headend to the subscriber. In coaxial cable systems, amplifiers are needed approximately every 1,500 feet. Amplifiers are also used in twisted copper pair telephone lines.

Analog - a continuously varying electrical signal in a shape of a wave. It is represented by continuous wave forms that vary in size and number as the source of the information varies. The variations in voice, loudness or pitch that a user hears at the other end reflects differences or fluctuations in the electrical current.

Asynchronous communication - two-way communication in which there is a time delay between when a message is sent and when it's received (e.g., electronic mail and voice mail).

Audiographic teleconferencing - refers to the transmission of graphic and text information over a narrowband telecommunications channel such as a telephone line or a sub-carrier.

Audio-teleconferencing - two way electronic voice communication between two or more people at two or more locations.

Backbone Network - a high speed transmission facility (e.g., optical fiber) designed to interconnect lower speed distribution channels.

Backhaul - a term used to describe the transmission of a signal (normally video) from the end of a microwave or broadcast system to a central point.

Bandwidth - a measure of the information carrying capacity of a communications channel; the higher the bandwidth, the greater the amount of information which can be carried.

Baud - a unit of digital transmission signalling speed of information transmission. It is used to describe the rate of information flow. Given in bits per second (bps) the rate is the highest number of single information elements (bits) transferred between two devices (such as modems or fax machines) in one second.

BBS (Bulletin Board Service) - a computer service that allows remote users to access a central "host" computer to read and post electronic messages.

Bit - stands for binary digit. It is the smallest possible unit of information making up a character or a word in digital code, and is represented as either "on" or "off" by the numbers "0" or "1." An electronic string of bits represents letters and symbols.

BITNET - The acronym for Because It's Time Network, an international electronic network. BITNET, privately owned by a consortium of U.S. colleges and universities, has about 2,500 host computers located primarily at universities.

Bridge - a device which is used to interconnect three or more telecommunications channels such as telephone lines, to permit simultaneous, two-way communication among all points which have been interconnected.

Broadband - communications which are capable of carrying a wide range of frequencies. Broadcast television, cable television, microwave, and satellite are examples of broadband technologies.

Cable television - a transmission system which distributes broadcast television signals and other services by means of coaxial cable. Residential cable subscribers are connected by means of cable to a central community antenna (CATV), which picks up signals from satellites for community distribution.

C-Band - a category of satellite transmission in the 6 GHz range. C-Band transmission generally requires a large antenna, or "downlink dish" because of its use of longer wavelength frequencies when compared to other transmission systems such as Ku-Band.

Central Office (Switching Office) - a local telephone company facility that houses the switching system and related equipment needed to interconnect telephone calls for customers in the immediate geographic area. Every LATA must have at least one central office.

Channel - a radio frequency assignment made according to the frequency band being used and the geographic location of the send/receive sites.

Coaxial cable - a metal cable consisting of a conductor in the form of a tube which can carry broadband signals by guiding high frequency electromagnetic signals. It is used for voice, data, and video.

Codec - a term used for a "code/decode" electrical device which converts an analog electrical signal into a digital form for transmission purposes. It is generally used to transform video signals into digital form for transmission over digital transmission systems. Generally speaking, this digital information must be reconverted into analog form at its point of reception.

Common carrier - A telecommunications company that is regulated by government agencies and offers communications relay services to the general public via shared circuits, charging published and non-discriminatory rates.

Compressed video - video images which have been processed to remove redundant information, reducing the amount of bandwidth needed to capture the necessary information so that the information can be sent over narrowband carriers such as a T1 telephone line

Computer conferencing - group communications through computers, or the use of shared computer files, remote terminal equipment and telecommunications channels for two-way, real-time group communication.

Conference call - a telephone call which, by making use of a bridge, connects more than two individuals at geographically distinct locations for simultaneous conversation.

CPR (Computed-based Patient Record) - the term for the computer-generated (electronic) patient record that is being developed.

Customer Premises Equipment (CPE) - devices ranging from simple telephones to computers to TV monitors that are located at a customer's location and are used to send or receive information over a telephone network.

Digital - discrete signals such as those represented by means of bits (which are either "on" or "off") as opposed to continuously variable analog signals. Used in both electronic and light-based systems, digital signals transmit audio, video, and data as bits. Digital technology allows communications signals to be compressed for more efficient transmission.

Direct Broadcast Satellite (DBS) - a satellite designed with sufficient power so that inexpensive earth stations, or downlinks, can be used for direct residential reception.

Direct Digital Imaging - involves the direct capture of digital images (e.g., an MRI) so that they can be electronically transmitted. This is in contrast to an x-ray that is first made into a film and then photographed for digitization to send or store.

Dish - a parabolic antenna that is the primary element of a satellite earth station, or downlink.

Downlink - the path, or link, from the satellite to earth stations which receive its signals. The term is frequently applied to a parabolic antenna that receives signals from a satellite. It is often referred to as: a dish, a terminal, an earth station, or a TVRO (television receive only).

DS1 - SEE T1

DS3 - SEE T3

Earth station - The ground equipment, including a dish and other electronics components needed to receive and/or transmit satellite telecommunications signals. An "uplink" is used for sending information to a satellite for distribution to various earth receiving stations, while a "downlink" is used to receive such information.

EDI (Electronic Data Interchange) - the sending and receiving of data directly between trading partners without paper or human intervention.

Equal Access - ability to choose between the different long distance carriers. In rural areas, some local exchange carriers are still serviced by only one long distance carrier.

Facsimile (Fax) - a device which electronically transmits and reproduces documents over telephone lines.

Fiber Optics - hair-thin, flexible glass rods encased in cables that use light to transmit audio, video, and data signals.

Footprint - the geographic region on the earth underneath a satellite which is in the appropriate range to receive that satellite's information.

Freeze frame - one method of transmitting still images over standard telephone lines. A single image is transmitted every 8-to-30 seconds. This is also referred to as slow scan.

Frequency - the rate at which an electromagnetic signal alternates. It is a term used with analog signals, and is reported in Hertz.

Full duplex - a communication channel over which both transmission and reception are possible in two directions at the same time. A standard telephone line is a full duplex system since people on either end of the connect can simultaneously speak while listening to sounds coming from the other end.

Full-motion video - a standard video signal that can be transmitted by a variety of means including television broadcast, microwave, fiber optics, and satellite. Full-motion video traditionally requires 6 MHz in analog format and 45 Mbps when encoded digitally.

Gb (Gigabit) - one billion bits of information - usually used to express a data transfer rate (e.g., 1 gigabit/second = 1Gbps). The bandwidth of optical fiber is often in the gigabit or billion-bits-per-second range.

Geostationary orbit - describes the orbit of a satellite whose position relative to the earth's surface is constant so it appears to hover over one spot on the earth's equator.

GHz (Gigahertz) - one billion cycles per second. It is a measurement of analog signal transmission.

Half duplex - a communication channel over which both transmission and reception are possible but only in one direction at a time.

HDTV (High Definition Television) - an advanced television system that produces video images as clear as high-quality photography.

Hertz - a unit of frequency equal to one cycle per second.

HPCC (High Performance Computing and Communications Program) - the HPCC initiative is a federal coordinated, interagency research and development effort designed to accelerate the availability and utilization of the next generation of high performance computers and networks.

Independent Telephone Company - a local exchange carrier that is not part of the Bell system of operating companies (BOCs). In rural areas, many of the independent telephone companies are cooperatives.

Informatics - the application of computer science and information science to the management and processing of data, information, and knowledge.

INTERNET - the largest international computer network. It is a network of computer networks linking computers from colleges and universities, government agencies, institutions, and commercial organizations worldwide. Owned by the U.S. government, it is used primarily for research and educational purposes.

ISDN (Integrated Services Digital Network) - a digital telecommunications channel that allows for the integrated transmission of voice, video, and data; a protocol for high-speed digital transmission. (see Table 2)

ITFS (Instructional Television Fixed Service) - a non-broadcast television service that is typically used for closed-circuit instructional applications. It requires special antennas and converters to translate signals for viewing.

IXC (Interexchange Carrier) - a telephone company such as AT&T, Sprint, or MCI that carries long distance calls. The IXCs are authorized by the FCC to carry interLATA, interstate traffic and can be authorized by state PUCs to carry interLATA, intrastate traffic. Also known as Long Distance Carriers.

Kbs - stands for kilobits (1000 bits) per second. It is a way of reporting the rate of transmission of digital information per second.

Ku-Band - frequencies in the 11-to-14 GHz band used to send and receive signals to and from satellites. Being somewhat more narrow than C-Band transmissions, the dish needed to receive these signals is smaller; Ku-Band tends to be somewhat less expensive than C-Band for this reason.

LANs (Local Area Networks) - data communication networks that are fairly limited in their reach - e.g., the premises of a building or a campus. They are private networks that facilitate the sharing of information and computer resources by the members of a group.

LATA - stands for Local Access Transport Area. These are local telephone service areas created by the divestiture of the regional Bell operating companies (RBOCs) formerly associated with AT&T.

LDC (Long Distance Carrier) - see IXC (Interexchange Carrier)

Leased lines - a line rented from a telephone company for the exclusive use of a customer. May also be called a dedicated line.

LEC (Local Exchange Carrier) - a telephone company that carries local calls.

Low-Altitude Satellites - satellites that orbit the Earth at lower altitudes than the geosynchronous satellites and cannot maintain a constant position above the Earth. Thus, they are only accessible when they come into view of the receiving dish, two or three times a day for a few minutes at a time.

Mbps - Megabits per second, or one million bits per second.

Medical informatics - the combination of computer science, information science, and the health sciences (medicine) designed to assist in the management and processing of data to support the delivery of health care.

Microwave - high frequency radio waves used for point-to-point communication of audio, video, and data signals. They can be simplex (omnidirectional) or duplex. The microwave spectrum is generally above 2 GHz. Microwave transmission requires line of sight transmission between sending and receiving antennas.

Modem - a modulator/demodulator. This device converts digital information into analog form for transmission over a telecommunications channel, and reconverts it to digital form at the point of reception.

Multiplexer - equipment which transmits two or more lines of voice, data, or video information over a single channel. For example, a multiplexer enables a single T1 telephone line to be split into a number of different "channels" to allow for multiple applications to be carried along the same T1 line.

Narrowband - a telecommunications medium, such as copper wire or part of a coaxial cable channel, that uses (relatively) low frequency signals. Generally speaking, narrowband transmissions go up to 1.544 Mbps.

Network - a set of nodes, points, or locations which are connected by means of data, voice, and video communications for the purpose of exchanging information.

NREN (National Research and Education Network) - the international, interconnected gigabit computer system network proposed under the HPCC initiative. The term "Interagency Interim NREN (IINREN) is now being used to describe the network.

NSFNET (National Science Foundation Network) - NSFNET is the high-speed network that connects mid-level regional computer (Internet) networks to support scientific research facilities throughout the country.

Packet Switching - the process of transmitting digital information by means of addressed packets - which include data, call control signals, and error control information - so that a channel is occupied only during the transmission of the packet. In contrast, data sent using modems occupies a circuit for the entire duration of the transmission, even when no data is actually traveling over the lines. Using packet switching, the various packets of information can travel along different routes on the network, allowing the carrier to optimize its network capacity.

PBX - stands for Private Branch Exchange, a computerized version of the telephone switchboard but with an expanded range of voice and data services. It operates as a private telephone exchange that serves a particular organization and has connections to the public telephone network.

POP (Point of Presence) - The point at which an interexchange carrier's circuits connect with local circuits for transmission and reception of long distance phone calls.

Port - a circuit in an electronic device for the input or output of signals.

PSTN (Public Switched Telephone Network) - the public telephone network.

Radio technology - used for telecommunications and broadcast services. Used for radio waves in frequencies that are distinct from those assigned to microwave services.

RANs (Rural Area Networks) - as conceptualized by the U.S. Congress, Office of Technology Assessment, RANs would be shared-usage networks, configured to include a wide range of users in rural communities - such as educational, health, and business entities.

RBOC (Regional Bell Operating Company) or Regional Holding Company - one of the seven regional companies formed by the AT&T divesture (Ameritech, Bell Atlantic, BellSouth, NYNEX, Pacific Telesis, Southwestern Bell and U.S. West. The BOCs (Bell Operating Companies) are grouped under the seven regional holding companies.

Repeater - a bi-directional device used in channels to amplify or regenerate signals.

RF - stands for radio frequency. Radio frequencies are electromagnetic signals which range from microwave to radio in length.

Routing - The assignment of a communication path by which a telephone call will reach its destination.

RS-232-C - A standard interface between a piece of equipment and a telephone circuit.

Rural Radio Service - the use of certain frequencies, distinct from those in microwave toll service, used to provide wireless telephony in rural areas. It can support the transmission of both analog and digital signals. It provides short-haul telecommunications, and requires different power, transmission, and reception capabilities and devices.

Satellite - an electronics retransmission device serving as a repeater, normally placed in orbit around the earth in geostationary orbit for the purpose of receiving and retransmitting electromagnetic signals. It normally receives signals from a single source and retransmits them over a wide geographic area, known as the satellite's "footprint."

Slow scan video - a device that transmits and receives still video pictures over a narrow telecommunications channel, such as standard telephone lines.

SMDS - (Switched Multimegabit Data Service) - SMDS is a high-speed, fast packet-switched service provided in a campus, or ring, type arrangement situated within a 50-mile radius.

SS7 (Signaling System 7) - a recent development in control systems for the public telephone network. It allows telephone company computers to communicate with each other, making telephone call processing faster and more efficient and enabling more services to be made available to consumers.

Switch - a mechanical or solid state device that opens or closes circuits, changes operating parameters, or selects paths or circuits on a space or time division basis.

Switched Network - a type of system where each user has a unique address (e.g., a phone number) which allows the network to connect any two points directly.

T1 (also known as DS1) - refers to a digital carrier capable of transmitting 1.544 Mbps of electronic information. It is the general term for a digital carrier available for high volume voice, data, or compressed video traffic. T1 is a standard for transmission that is accepted in North America. **Fractional T1 or sub T1** tariffs are rates for bandwidths between 56 Kbps and 1.544Mbps, such as 384Kbps = 1/2 a T1.

T3 (also known as DS3) - a carrier of 45 Mbps bandwidth. One T3 channel can carry 28 T1 channels.

T-carrier - a series of transmission systems using pulse code modulation technology at various channel capacities and bit rates to send digital information over telephone lines, including optical fiber lines, or another transmission medium.

Telecommunications - the use of wire, radio, optical, or other electromagnetic channels to transmit or receive signals for voice, data, and video communications.

Teleconferencing - interactive electronic communication between two or more people at two or more sites which make use of voice, video, and/or data transmission systems: audio, audiographics, computer, and video systems.

Telemedicine - the use of telecommunications for medical diagnosis and patient care.

Teletext - a broadcasting service using several otherwise unused scanning lines (vertical blanking intervals) between frames of TV pictures to transmit information from a central database to receiving television sets.

Terrestrial Carrier - a telecommunications transmission system using land-based facilities (microwave towers, telephone lines, coaxial cable, fiber optic cable) as distinguished from satellite transmission.

Translator - a broadband network operation. A translator is a device which is located in a central retransmission facility to filter incoming microwave signals and retransmit them in a higher frequency band.

Transmission Speed - the speed at which information passes over the line; defined in either bits per second (bps) or baud.

Transponder - a microwave repeater (receiver and transmitter) in a satellite that receives signals being sent from earth, amplifies them, and sends them back down to earth for reception purposes. Domestic communication satellites use either 12 or 24 transponders, equivalent to a single channel, which usually have a 36 MHz bandwidth.

Trunk - a large capacity, long distance channel used by common carriers to transfer information between its customers.

Turn-key system - a telecommunications system in which all components and installation services needed for operational teleconferencing have been provided by a single vendor or contractor.

TVRO (Television Receive Only) - an earth station capable of receiving satellite TV signals but not of transmitting them; a "downlink."

Twisted Pair - cable made of a pair of insulated copper wires wrapped around each other to cancel the effects of electrical noise. It can transmit voice and data and, in some cases, low-grade video. It is the most prevalent type of medium in PSTN's local loops. The wire-pair sizes typically range from 19-to-26 gauge. Cables with as many as 2,700 pairs of 26-gauge wire are used in urban areas.

Uplink - the path, or link, from a transmitting earth station tothe satellite. The term is frequently applied to a transmitting earth station.

Voice grade channel - a telephone circuit of sufficient bandwidth to carry signals in the voice frequency range of 300-to-3400 Hertz.

Voice Switching - an electrical technique for opening and closing a circuit, such as changing from one microphone to another microphone or from one video camera to another video camera, in response to the presence or absence of sound.

VSAT (Very Small Aperture Terminal) - a type of satellite dish (1.8-2.4 meters in diameter). Used primarily for data transmissions (low speed to high speed). Can send and receive voice, data and video signals if enhanced. VSATs can transmit over wide areas by relaying to satellites in geosynchronous orbit.

WANs (Wide Area Networks) - data communication networks that provide long-haul connectivity among separate networks located in different geographic areas.

WATS (Wide Area Telephone Service) - a flat rate or measured bulk rate long distance service provided on an incoming or outgoing basis. WATS permits a customer, by use of an access line, to make telephone calls to any dial-able telephone number in a specific zone for a flat or bulk monthly rate using an 800 number.

References:

Dillon, C., Blanchard, D., Price, M. (1989). *The Emerging Role of Telecommunications in Higher Education: A Teleconference Resource Book*. Norman: University of Oklahoma.

Hedblom, H., and Spurr, M. (1989). *Wiring Minnesota: New State Goals for Telecommunications*. Minneapolis, MN: Citizens League.

Oregon ED-Net, Portland, OR.

Parker, E. & Hudson, H. (1992) *Electronic Byways*. Boulder, CO:Westview Press, Inc.

Schmidt and Smith (in press) *Telemedicine: The Role of Telemedicine in Health Care Delivery*. Topeka, KS: Kansas Hospital Association and Kansas Department of Health and Environment.

Stallings, W. (1989). *ISDN: An Introduction*. New York: MacMillan.

U. S. Congress, Office of Technology Assessment (OTA), U.S. Congress. 1989. *Linking for Learning: A New Course for Education*. Washington, DC: U.S. Government Printing Office.

U. S. Congress, Office of Technology Assessment (OTA), U.S. Congress. 1991. *Rural America at the Crossroads: Networking for the Future*. Washington, DC: U.S. Government Printing Office.

U. S. Department of Commerce, National Telecommunications and Information Administration. 1991. *The NTIA Infrastructure Report: Telecommunications in the Age of Information*. Washington, DC: U.S. Department of Commerce.

TABLE 1

Transmission Channels

Channel	Bandwidth/ Transmission Speeds	
Twisted-pair Copper	4KHz (64Kbps) *	One twisted copper pair transmitting at 4KHz can carry 48 calls. It originally required a 64Kbps channel to send a digitized voice call; today a voice grade call can require as little as 8Kbps to 16 Kbps. A conventional 3" thick cable contains 1,200 pairs of copper wires.
Co-axial Cable	140 Mbps	Coaxial cable consists of up to 22 coaxial conductors. (A coaxial conductor is a copper tube as big around as a pencil; a copper wire is held in the tube's center by plastic insultators.) Coaxial cable is used to transmit video, voice and data. A pair of coaxial tubes can carry up to 13,200 telephone calls. Cable TV systems use coaxial cable to carry TV signals into subscribers' homes. Some TV networks use coaxial cable to send their programs to affiliated stataions for broadcasting to viewers. Coaxial cable is also used in LANS. Coaxial cable is capable of carrying two-way signals, but most systems are currently designed for uni-directional use.
Optical Fiber		Optical fiber is used by telephone companies for long distance trunk lines and by cable TV companies to carry TV signals into the homes of subscribers.
	565 Mbps	565 Mbps is a commonly used optical fiber transmission speed. At 565 Mbps a single fiber pair can carry more than 8,000 voice channels. Ninety-six fibers (or 48 fiber pairs) can carry more than 384,000 voice channels.
	1.2 Gbps	At 1.2 Gbps, a single fiber pair can carry 18,816 voice channels.
	1.7 Gbps	At 1.7 Gbps, a single fiber pair can carry 24,192 voice channels.
	3.4 Gbps	3.4 Gbps is the fastest commercial transmission speed available in the early 1990s.
Microwave Relay Systems +		Microwaves, a type of electromagnetic wave, are short, super high frequency radio waves that travel in straight lines. Microwave systems can transmit either analog or digital signals. Commercial terrestrial fixed microwave systems operate at frequencies between 1.7 GHz and 23 GHz. The amount of bandwidth available varies from system to system.
	45 Mbps	Some phone company microwave systems use 45 Mbps channels. This is equivalent to 28 T1 circuits or channels.
Microwave ITFS	6MHz per channel in the 2.5 GHz band	Instructional Television Fixed Service is a special band of the microwave frequencies reserved for educational purposes by the FCC.

Radio Relay Systems	AM band - 535-1705 KHz FM band - 88-108 MHz	Radio waves, used for radio and TV broadcasting and for telecommunications, are high frequency electromagnetic waves that are longer than microwaves. They can transmit either analog or digital signals. Radio broadcasting waves follow the curve of the earth, in contrast to microwaves which travel in straight lines. Frequencies assigned for use by radio systems are distinct from those assigned to microwave toll service. The AM band of frequencies ranges from 535 - 1705 KHz; the FM band from 88 - 108 MHz. A single FM radio channel may require only 150 KHz; an AM channel only 10 KHz.
Digital	180 Mbps	A digital radio system used for telecommunications is capable of transmitting 4 DS-3 channels or 180 Mbps.
Satellite	C: 4GHz/6GHz Ku: 12GHz/14GHz Ka: 30 GHz/20GHz	Satellites function as relay stations in the sky -- satellite transponders receive signals from an uplink and transmit them back to Earth. The transponders generally operate in two frequency bands: C-band and Ku-band. Until recently, most transponders had a 36MHz bandwidth and could transmit 6 TV broadcast channels of 6MHz each. With new compression technologies, transponders can carry more channels. The C or Ku band GHz/GHz designation refers to the frequency bands in which signals are transmitted, not to the bandwidth of the signals being transmitted. For example, in the Ku-band, the channel bandwidth used to transmit analog video signals might range from 34-54 MHz. Ka-band is the newest of these technology.
Terrestrial Broadcast Systems for Television	6 MHz analog or 45 Mbps digital	TV signals are electromagnetic waves that fall within the radio frequency spectrum. TV signals consist of modulated video and audio carrier waves. TV signals can be received clearly up to a distance of 75 - 150 miles; to be sent further, they must be converted to microwaves. The group of frequencies over which one TV station broadcasts is known as a channel. 68 channels are available in the United States and Canada; Channels 2-13 are VHF channels (very high frequency) and Channels 14-69 are UHF channels (ultrahigh frequency). A TV channel broadcasting in analog occupies a band of frequencies that is 6MHz wide.
High Definition Television (HDTV)	1.3 Gbps	High Definition Television (HDTV) is an advanced television system that produces video images as sharp as high-quality photographs. Work is underway to develop compression technology to enable HDTV to be transmitted by a bandwidth of 6 MHz.

* The actual capacity of twisted copper pair will vary with distance. That is, it varies directly with gauge and inversely with distance such that a 24 gauge twisted pair copper wire can carry 1.5 Mbps of traffic to about 6 feet or 2.4 Kbps to about 10 miles.

\+ Radio frequency bands range from 15KHz to 300GHz. Within this, the microwave frequency bands range from 300MHz to 300GHz.

TABLE 2

Compression Standards and Comparisons

1 bit - 1 b	- Binary digit. The smallest possible unit of information making up a character or a word in digital code, represented either as "on" or "off" by the numbers "0" or "1."
1,000 bits - 1 Kbps	- *one thousands bits per second or a kilobit/second*
56,000 bits - 56 Kbps	- Compressed video can be transmitted at 56 Kbps. 56 Kbps is sometimes offered on a "dial-up" basis.
64,000 bits - 64 Kbps	- DS-0 capacity. 64 Kbps or DS-O is the basis of a digital channel.
384,000 bits - 384 Kbps	- 1/4 of a T1 channel or a "fractional T1" or a "sub-T1." Using new codecs meeting a new international standard, quality compressed video can be transmitted at this speed.
1,000,000 bits - 1 Mbps	- *one million bits per second or a megabit/second*
1,544,000 bits - 1.54 Mbps	- T1 or DS-1 capacity. This is a common transmission speed for compressed interactive video. It is also the transmission standard for Primary ISDN.
2,140,000 bits - 2.14 Mbps	- The transmission speed of optical fiber in 1978.
45,000,000 bits - 45 Mbps	- T3 or DS-3 capacity. This transmission speed supports full motion video and is used in telemedicine applications such as fluoroscopy.
155,000,000 bits - 155 Mbps	- The transmission speed for ATM (Asynchronous Transfer Mode) or fast packet switching.
274,000,000 bits - 274 Mbps	- T4 or DS-4 capacity.
545,000,000 bits - 545 Mbps	- The common transmission speed for commercial optical fiber. At 545 Mbps a single fiber pair can carry 8,000 voice channels.
1,000,000,000 bits - 1 Gbps	- *one billion bits per second or a gigabit/second*
1,300,000.000 bits - 1.3 Gbps	- HDTV requirements without compression.
2,000,000,000 bits - 2 Gbps	- The transmission speed of optical fiber speed in 1990.
3,400,000,000 bits - 3.4 Gbps	- The fastest commercial transmission speed for optical fiber in the early 1990s.

Compression Standards and Comparisons (cont.)

T or DS Transmission Standards

Bandwidth capacity can be designated by using standards, e.g. T1. These standards indicate how much information can be transmitted per second over the channel. It is helpful to recognize that a T1 "channel" is not necessarily an actual physical conduit or line, such as a cable, but is an amount of information that can be transferred per second by a range of telecommunications circuits or channels. For example, T1 amounts of information can be transmitted over wireline channels (i.e., enhanced twisted copper pair, co-axial cable, optical fiber) or over radio wave channels using digital radio or terrestrial microwave or satellite.

DS-0	= 64,000 bits per second (64 Kbps).	This is the basis of all digital network standards.
T1 or DS-1	= 1,544,000 bits per second (1.544Mbps).	This is 24 64Kbps channels (23 for audio, video and data; 1 for signalling; and 8000 bits for framing.)
T2 or DS-2	= 6,300,000 bits per second (6.3Mbps).	
T3 or DS-3	= 45,000,000 bits per second (45Mbps).	This provides full-motion video for telemedicine applications and is the speed of Switched Multimegabit Data Service (SMDS).

ISDN Protocols or Transmission Standards

Like T carrier standards, ISDN designations are also standards or protocols that have been agreed upon for transferring information over channels. (Protocols are agreed upon standards that allow devices to communicate with each other.) Standards for ISDN are being established by the Consultative Committee for International Telephone and Telegraph (CCITT). All of the standard ISDN interfaces are based on a multiple of a digital voice grade channel - i.e., 64 Kbps. ISDN standards vary internationally; in Europe primary ISDN is 30 64Kbps channels and 1 64Kbps signalling channel. ISDN systems require digital input and output devices.

ISDN Basic Service	= 144 Kbps	= 2 64Kbps channels + 1 16Kbps channel for signalling. [2B + 1D]
ISDN Primary Service	= 1.544 Kbps	= 23 64Kbps channels + 1 64Kbps channel for signalling (equivalent of T1). [23B + 1D]
ISDN Broadband Service	= (150Mbps)	Dynamically configurable channels at rates up to 150 Mbps using optical fiber. The broadband standards are under discussion, with 45 Mbps serving as an interim standard.

Mr. HAYES. There are a few things I am interested in. One goes back to one of Gary's earlier statements about the difference between legislation and its impact in the instance in which you spoke in rural America.

I often try to tell people at home that if you are diagramming a play, it is great to go to a meeting before a football game and watch a play diagrammed because it is always going to work on the blackboard. In real life when you watch the University of Southern California run the student body left, the right tackle kicks the left corner. That means about a 300-pound person is quicker than most track athletes at most major universities, will probably be a first-round draft choice, and as long as that is what you have running the play, it is going to work. When instead you have a 160-pound person who is trying to line up with a 250-pound defensive end from Notre Dame, it is going to fail.

The point that I am making is that in much of the health care system, and that is why I am so glad you came today and Dr. Sanders came today, the realities of who is playing at what position affect the framework and have to be thought of in advance. In this field of telemedicine, certainly the fiscal capabilities, the financial capabilities, are absolutely real, and we can diagram this afternoon a perfect system in theory for Cameron Parish, Louisiana. In practice we are going to have to pay for it and then we are going to have to also figure out where we find the people that we just magically assume are going to run different parts and elements of it. That I think is an unintended consequence.

As you were speaking, as both you and Dr. Sanders were speaking, I got to thinking about the earlier testimony from the other Dr. Sanders who said that we should look at the system as if it is a visit from the patient to the physician crossing State lines, and I wondered if those who wrote the language, for example, in some of the health care plans, not just the President's, but others, who talk about not going distances for treatment ever thought that the legal theory might be that you went somewhere whether you left the house or not, and you end up with a competition, which Gary mentioned, of those who want to compete for their own economic interests suddenly arguing that you can't do something even though it was never intended that that language prohibit an act from taking place. And almost every regulatory scheme I deal with, whether it is environmental or whether it is medical or anything else, usually ends up with the unintended consequence being the biggest problem, rather than the actual issue that was being addressed.

If you were to design it, I am curious, from Dr. Sanders' point of view, if you were to design in cooperation with Beaumont or Galveston or Lake Charles, wherever, what would be the basic—in the field we are talking about, teleconferencing, telecommunications, what would be the basic things that would be most important and why—in other words, with all these choices that Gary is talking about being thrust upon you, what would be the things that would lead you to have to say what you would go to the parish and try to be in favor of having to financially support?

What criteria would you use in trying to say, one, what you need, and two, how to make a choice as to different and competing entities that are trying to convince you what you need from their standpoint, their economic interest standpoint.

Dr. RICHARD SANDERS. The first thing with the entities of course is going to be the cost, how much they charge the hospital. That was another thing. I think that any cost that is going to the individual hospitals, they are indigent care—I am dealing quite a bit with the indigents, and just people that just are on subsistence salaries. The hospitals should not be required to bear the cost of telecommunication for these people. I think it ought to be one all-inclusive charge for the hospital or something, but not for each individual patient.

But the main criteria that I would use about this would be how quickly I could get the consultant when I need him. For instance, if it is the middle of the night and I have a myocardial infarction, the guy's blood pressure is dropping and I am calling the cardiologist and they are saying, Wait a minute, we are going to find him and it is going to take him 30 minutes to get on the phone or take him 30 minutes to be able to consult with me, really and truly I am back in the situation, I am flying by the seat of my pants or I am using my own judgment on this. That would be the number one criteria, I feel. And number two would be the cost involved of the system to the hospital, to the parish.

Mr. HAYES. Be interested, Gary, you wanted to make any comment on that? Because you had brought up the point earlier of those competitive forces. I would imagine—I would imagine from the experience you gave, you might want to add something from the standpoint of how you think local and rural physicians are going to have to deal with the decision-making process.

Mr. RAVETTO. I think that they should—the ultimate decision should be left there. The scenario that you just described and Dr. Sanders commented on is the ideal one, and that is that the opportunities, both financial for the equipment and the establishment—and the maintenance of the network be brought to that local community and let the local community decide what is best for itself, as opposed to, what I get the sense tends to happen sometimes, and that is the larger institutions or the bureaucracies on the State level at least come in and say, this is how it is going to be.

I don't want to sound over-critical of them. In many cases, it is with the best of intentions, but the reality is there are many, many other factors, as you had alluded to, that play into every community.

I mean, Dr. Sanders, as you know, he is the only doctor in that parish. The hospital is a relatively strong hospital, but the community—the population is different than other communities that you go north in Louisiana, particularly go to Bernice that only has one doctor, has a failing hospital, has a very—equal population size, but very different problems, so therefore they have to solve them in a very different way.

So I think that—I hope I am answering your question. I think that ultimately the decision should be left to the community with some kind of regulations and some kind of quality control, if you will, but still they should be able to decide for themselves, and ultimately, and I have said this to rural hospitals all the time, if they and their communities are not committed to having a strong health care system in their own community, then they have no one else to blame but themselves when the local facility closes or the doctor leaves. It has to be something that a community wants.

I think, particularly in Louisiana, rural America has sat back and expected the powers that be to solve their problems for them. Then they have sat in judgment of whether you all have done the right thing or not. And that just doesn't work and it hasn't worked. They have to empower themselves to solve their problems. I think you can give them the tools to do that or the opportunities but they have to do it for themselves.

Mr. HAYES. Secondly, we haven't talked about this today and, Dena, you obviously would have maybe a greater aforethought to it, but one of the things I was wondering in sitting here listening through this part as it involves the health care industry is, how do you impose the concept of gatekeeper in telemedicine?

In other words, do they have to phone or find someone else at 3:00 in the morning that is in effect approving your call to whomever you found is going to give you hopefully some assistance in an emergency procedure? At all the meetings and conferences you have probably been to, I would like to know if that has ever been discussed, and if so, in what context and with what thoughts toward resolution.

Dr. PUSKIN. Yes, it has been discussed. I don't think it has been resolved but it has certainly been discussed. Let me just say, there are two issues in terms of gatekeeper. In the context of a capitated system, it is less of an issue because there is no incentive to just willy-nilly use telemedicine—the financial incentive isn't there.

The concern is in fee-for-service, where the incentive might be—some have said, just to walk the patient by the screen, one after another, to generate a lot of revenues. I think that is an extreme, but there may be less judiciousness in how to use it.[1]

The reality of the systems that are operating now is that the consultations have to be scheduled and that, in fact, it is not that easy just to call up for a consult. In the systems that exist now, there are some natural controls on the availability and use of telemedicine.

I think one of the reasons for more demonstrations that are widespread and more systems out there that we have information on is to basically look and see what some of the gatekeeper issues may be and how to best do that.

In the systems I have looked at to date, I don't see a lot of abuse. There are people worried about the potential for abuse of the system to generate revenues. I haven't seen it to date because, as I said, the.[2] But I wouldn't say it couldn't happen. I think part of the way you get around that is to bring telemedicine into system of care.

When doctors like Dr. Sanders call for an emergency consultation, there is no question that telemedicine is advisable. The question comes when practitioners schedule clinics, run 50 patients

[1] Dr. Puskin wants to add "under a fee-for-service system."
[2] Dr. Puskin wants to add "need to schedule consults has precluded overuse."

through[3,4] and you say, Ha, ha, and you charge it off to third-party payers. This is a possibility but I don't think it is going to become an over whelming concern because people have already begun to think about how to set up utilization controls for it.

Mr. HAYES. Thanks. I turn it over to Ms. Morella.

Mrs. MORELLA. I thank the panel.

I feel very responsible having you here, particularly Dr. Sanders. What if there is a medical emergency in your parish?

Dr. RICHARD SANDERS. Absolutely. We have hired a physician. You can hire temporary physicians to fill in for you. We have hired one. He is going to be sitting there until I get home tonight. I am sorry. Excuse me.

Mrs. MORELLA. Relieved to hear that.

Mr. Ravetto, you said something about this would be a good tool for recruiting and retaining primary care physicians. Would you explain how it would be?

Mr. RAVETTO. Well, one of the issues that we face regularly in trying to recruit young physicians and also relocate practicing physicians is this idea of isolation, professional isolation, and if you think about the fact that professionally you have colleagues that you interact with on a regular basis, face to face, and you can share ideas and talk, look at Dr. Sanders. He is the only physician within—closest one is 40 some miles, almost 50 miles away. There is that professional isolation. There is no way for him to communicate and to share ideas and to stay mentally stimulated and do all those things to keep him healthy professionally and personally and happy and successful.

I think that this is an important link that will do that. It is not the ideal. The ideal is people touching people, but I think this is as close as we can get to it. It will give him the opportunity, and fellow doctors like him, the opportunity to talk with each other and to communicate and to share patients so that he won't feel as isolated, as alone, and hopefully then it will encourage more young people to choose a rural practice and ultimately primary care.

Mrs. MORELLA. It would be interesting at a medical school that deals with particularly rural physician training to find out if, in fact, that would enhance that kind of long distance communication, and it probably would.

I have always been curious in something that was mentioned, how you did the billing, how you would do the billing, since cost is—what Dr. Puskin said was such a major factor, whether you—you know, as you say, whether they walk by the screen for the examination, whether it is through your telephone. You, particularly dealing with rural areas, would have a greater problem in terms of how this would be facilitated.

Dr. PUSKIN. Well, there is only one place right now where at least Medicare and Medicaid are paying for it, and that is in Georgia, in Jay Sanders' project and it gets billed as a visit. And in Jay's project—and, Jay, correct me if I am wrong—the physicians at both ends are getting paid, which is one model.

[3] Dr. Puskin wants to add "who may not need specialty consults, and."
[4] Dr. Puskin wants to delete "and you say ha, ha, and you"

But I think what is of interest, and what I think HCFA hopes to do more of, and I don't know if Helen touched upon this, is looking at some of the alternative ways for third parties pay for telemedicine consults and some of the pros and cons of those alternatives. Because clearly fee-for-service, as I said, is really the issue here, and we have different options for how to pay for this.

We could pay essentially a sort of—set up a global contract and, you know, you get—Dr. Sanders here could contract with a medical school and get essentially in, for that amount he gets a certain amount of consultations and he gets billed in some kind of—the network gets billed a global amount to support everyone who participates, as has been discussed, and there are multiple ways of doing it.

The fact is, we haven't begun to really explore payment options in a way that allows us to figure out what are both the positive and the negative incentives in each. There is a lot of concern, as has been mentioned here, that telemedicine will promote utilization. Some of that is just expected. You are going to begin to treat and give people services who didn't get them before.

It is not surprising that this might raise costs. The question becomes, what are your offsetting savings as offsets, and how do you best set up a system for allow for billing that doesn't create inordinate incentives for abuses, and I don't think we have explored that. And that is, I think, why a lot of people are saying, We need to expand what we are doing in terms of programs like Jay's, but we might not want to open payment right now to everyone.

Dr. RICHARD SANDERS. Representative Morella, this is interesting, the University of Texas in Houston approximately 12 years ago set up a toll-free number where any physician could call and ask any question he wants to, whichever specialist he would like, and this is totally on the telephone. It was set up primarily at the University of Texas so Herman Hospital could get referrals. They set it up and it has been very profitable for them.

For example, over the last 12 years, I have sent them approximately 30 different referrals for them, so it actually can be profitable for the hospital that is on the receiving end of these transmissions if they are receiving referrals.

Now, obviously if I am receiving, or Mayo clinic is receiving a transmission from me, they are not going to get a referral when they are in Minnesota and I am in Louisiana, but in some instances, for instance, in Houston they could. Or if they are in New Orleans at Auschner or at LSU Medical Center or something, they could receive a referral there.

Dr. PUSKIN. West Virginia University prior to their new M.D. TV project, which we are funding there, also had for many years a telephone consultation service. It cost them about $100,000 a year. In Alabama, they also have a successful telephone referral system, which certainly says that it is probably cost effective for the institution, but it doesn't say whether, in the end, this is going to attract physicians to widespread participation in these systems. And I think the issue is physician reimbursement.

Mrs. MORELLA. Right, right. Indeed. Dr. Sanders mentioned the need for really making it multilingual too.

Dr. RICHARD SANDERS. Correct.

Mrs. MORELLA. I can see there will be a tremendous need for that. We worked on the multilingual, toll-free, around-the-clock hotline for domestic violence. Indeed, there could be something ultimately set up to make sure it is multilingual.

You mentioned that you would still need the rural physician. I agree with you, but on the other hand, since you have so few, you could also use the other practitioners, couldn't you? You could use even nurses aides and nurse practitioners, et cetera.

Dr. PUSKIN. Yes. If I use the word physician, I meant to use the word practitioner.

Mrs. MORELLA. Maybe you did. I think Dr. Sanders was saying we still need rural practitioners.

Dr. PUSKIN. Which would cover nurse practitioners and physician assistants. I think the fear in rural communities when I speak to them—and I speak a lot to them—is that somehow we are going to use telemedicine as a way of not providing the kind of incentives and efforts for getting rural practitioners out there. We have a lot of programs that we are talking about expanding now, like the National Health Service Corps, and similar State programs to get practitioners out there. There is a fear that we will lose sight of that and the need for these programs and use telemedicine as an excuse. And that local communities and States, in particular, will see this as a way not to continue their efforts in the areas of building incentive systems for physicians and nurse practitioners.

I think there is a real fear there. Whether it is realistic or not, the fear is real.

Mr. RAVETTO. If I may underscore what you just said, you are absolutely correct in that and I think that one could say that it goes as far as saying it is a very large fear that communities have. They really feel that they have been under siege for a long time economically. The comment that was made earlier about the interstate system in this country and what it did to rural America, maybe that started it. I don't know.

But there is a fear out there that those of us who make decisions for them on their behalf are—somehow have this—we are intentionally out there trying to let them—or encourage them to wither away, and there is a perception that a community needs a hospital, they need a doctor. Whether it is correct or not, it is the perception. It is what they believe. They need a church, they need a school system. And I have got myself in some problems locally, about six or eight months ago because I was asked to address the idea—in fact, it was something that we did with Congressman Hayes about the idea of nurse practitioners, and I said that we support them and we encourage them, however, I don't know how accepting they will be in many rural communities because as the leadership there looks for economic viability to try to keep those communities alive, the idea of having a doctor in that town or doctors is extremely important to them, and I don't know whether that is necessarily wrong.

Maybe it is too naive to think that we can continue to do that and maybe we are wasting time and money and energy in trying to do it. But again, maybe I am too idealistic. Ultimately, I would like to see that. I think it is a very important component to the health, not only the physical health, but the social health of those communities that they exist.

Dr. PUSKIN. Could I just say something about integrated systems of care and what we envision? We don't think every community, especially very small frontier communities, will be able to have and support a physician full-time. I think there are some realities that we have to deal with, and it will depend on the community. There are lots of variations. But, by broadening your view of the health care system from this little community here and another little community, but a group of communities that work together and are part of a system of care that is responsible for ensuring that the residents of that care—of that community get care. For example there may be a small clinic in one community that is run by a nurse practitioner, which is—that clinic is affiliated with a nearby clinic that is affiliated with a larger medical center. And the referral relationships are set up such that telemedicine serves as a tool for communication and linkage among all those practitioners who provide an on-site presence of care.

And it may be that the way we organize our care system may allow us to have services in communities that right now are in serious danger of losing all their services. We need to to look at alternatives so that that hospital that closes, because it cannot survive for whatever reason, may, in fact, become a good ambulatory clinic, which it probably already is largely an ambulatory clinic, and that if it is linked appropriately, so the practitioners no longer feel the professional isolation, then that community and its residents will have access to the best services available.

And telemedicine can help that as an adjunct and a linkage to insure that those practitioners are backed up.

Mr. RAVETTO. I don't mean to turn this into a debate but I really—and I don't disagree with what you are saying, but I think the political realities of it is, and looking at Congressman Hayes, he can tell you going out there that he certainly would not want to go out to any of the communities in the district he serves and say to them, We have decided, whomever has decided, that you are the community that is not going to have a doctor. These are towns that have vacant storefronts. They are ghost towns.

Mrs. MORELLA. They don't have a doctor now.

Mr. RAVETTO. Some do. But what I am saying is that it is a challenge to be able to be in that decision—I am not disagreeing with it. Actually I agree very much. I think that is the reality. But it is taking the reality and taking it out to those people and trying to explain to them that this is what is going to happen.

Dr. PUSKIN. I don't want to turn it into a debate either, but my view is that some of those communities will have doctors, and in others, they will have to come to some other decisions. And they are part of that decision making process.

Mr. HAYES. Again, I want to jump back in in the questioning. I think that part of this, if we went all the way back to our very first witness today, is in the definition of community. In the language that Gary and Dr. Sanders and I are speaking of in Dr. Sanders' parish, Creole and Cameron were never going to have competing hospitals and Johnson Bayou was not going to be concerned that it didn't have a doctor in Johnson Bayou. Yet I just named three communities from a geopolitical standpoint from a governmental organization, and I think perhaps the correct phrase we ought to be using is community of interest, because if there is not anyone in Creole, Johnson Bayou, Cameron, collectively, and there is not a presence, that is a community of interest that feels quite different, and because of the diversity of rural America, the examples that would come to my mind would be probably dramatically different than those of you in many other States and in rural America as represented by them.

But I think that is really what Gary is saying more, is within that community of interest, and within that community of interest, it might be saleable to say that this township as organized by government does not have a doctor, but if we expand that to mean this group of people that are somewhat homogenous, even though they cross some political lines, does not have a doctor, that has quite a different meaning.

So I am not sure that we are saying something that is so different if our definition of terms were to become the same, because I don't think we could sell a health care program, nor by the way would I care to try to sell one that removes a local community of interest. But it certainly is not—to reverse that, I wouldn't care to go out and try to sell a health plan that promised every political subdivision is going to have direct access to a physician. I think we just have to create the balance and realize where those community interests are.

Dr. RICHARD SANDERS. Excuse me for interrupting. It is not that the primary care physician is going to replace the emergency room. In any area you go to, it is very reassuring to know that you have an emergency room. If an emergency arises for yourself, your children, et cetera, you have got someplace you can go to in the middle of the night, et cetera. It is not going to replace that, but it will enhance it.

Mrs. MORELLA. Is the Federal program of scholarships for a medical school for service in rural or needy areas, is that working? We hear many stories about it.

Mr. RAVETTO. I will have to start first. It is an area that I feel very strong. I don't think that it is, quite frankly. And I don't mean to get into a debate on that topic, but we see students who come down through the National Health Service Corps or other programs who are from other places in the country and who are placed in our area and they don't stay. There are strong cultural differences. Some of it is the community's fault because they are not welcoming, but some of it is just very natural.

A quick story. When I was up in Washington the end of January and the first of February, I ran into a lady who was with the American Medical Association and she told me that she was leaving her office in Chicago one evening and a phone call came in and she just happened to grab the phone before she left and it was a doctor who was through the National Health Service Corps that was from New York City, a black gentleman, who was placed in a very small, very Southern, very stereotypical white community in Georgia, and he was ready to commit suicide that night. And she told the story to me and she said he hated it. He couldn't wait to get out. He felt like he was sold back into slavery. He felt it was the worst thing that ever happened to him.

She fortunately got the State medical society president on the phone. While she had him on hold, he found the local county president of the medical society and the gentleman went over and spent the evening with him and talked him through it. That is an extreme, and when she told me, I really thought she was exaggerating.

But the reality of it is, I think that in some of the matches they aren't taking into account the fact that in southwest Louisiana, a lot of the older people speak Cajun French. They are not welcoming of outsiders. They don't want to undress in front of someone that they feel is not like them.

And that is true in Western Pennsylvania where I grew up. My grandmother was very indignant about the fact that there was a foreign doctor who was going to examine her in the rural community she lived in.

Those are some of the realities. I think that if it could match people more culturally, they could have a tendency to stay. That is not at least what I see happening in the part of the State that I serve.

Dr. RICHARD SANDERS. Excuse me. When I was in medical school, I was kind of in the post–Vietnam era right after the draft ended and the military was needing physicians desperately, so it began offering a health scholarship program, scholarships in which you would serve a year in the military for each year they put you through medical school, and you kind of have to look at the scholarship programs that go to underserved areas like that. They are designed only as a stop-gap measure.

I was in the Air Force but only for two-and-a-half years by the time they put me through medical school, whereas you have other physicians, very good, excellent physicians, well recognized, world renowned such as Dr. Gomez who stayed in and made a career out of it; the majority of us got out after our time was over with. That is kind of the way the scholarship program is right now. They are going to do two years, four years, whatever the commitment is, and they are going to move on somewhere else.

Dr. PUSKIN. I think the history of the National Health Service Corps has been very mixed. There certainly is an attempt, whenever possible to match, but that doesn't always work, in part because you don't have the matches. It becomes a—certainly becomes a problem. Many people—you know, they serve out their tour of duty and then move on.

Interestingly enough, sometimes they move from one rural community to another. So one thing you have achieved is at least they are serving a rural community. It may not be the one that they were placed in, but the physicians and other practitioners who might not have thought about rural practice are now at least in rural practice.

And I don't have the figures here, but they can be provided. I think about 20 percent but I am not entirely stay within a reasonable area of where they were placed. As I said, I don't have the exact figures.

But the point is that people do move on in life. We often don't keep the first job that we had. How many of us are in the same job and live in the same place as our first job? I think that is something to be kept in mind about the realities of the age of these people and what happens in our mobile society.

The question is, over time, is this the only answer for meeting our health care needs in these communities? No, there are a lot of other solutions that we would like to have. One of those solutions is to build a system of health care to support, attract and retain people so they want to come to rural communities. And you want to train them appropriately for rural practice. All these elements have to come in place, and the National Health Service Corps is only one piece.

In my opinion, we have not put it all together yet and part of what we need to do is put it all together.

Mrs. MORELLA. Good point. The National Health Service Program, it sounds like it should also do some screening at the very beginning.

Dr. PUSKIN. And they are increasingly sensitive to that, but it does not work all the time.

Mrs. MORELLA. Just a final point. I was reading a number of the publications that we have from you, Dr. Puskin. I appreciate very much, but you do mention a rural outreach program with the National Library of Medicine.

I wonder if you might want to explain how you link up with it, and whether Dr. Sanders and Mr. Ravetto want to comment on it. I guess it is the Grateful Med?

Dr. PUSKIN. Right, actually the National Library of Medicine has a number of programs that I thought, in reading Don Lindberg's testimony, he may have mentioned. Grateful Med is a literature—enables physicians like Dr. Sanders to access through their personal computer, a full range of the medical literature so that they have access to the Library of Medicine no matter where they are.

And the library, it is my understanding, has a number of outreach programs that they have instituted around the country, to basically reach out to rural communities and make information more accessible on health care.

We have a rural health outreach grant program. Since we have put out so many publications, I am not quite sure, in which we basically have funded some telemedicine projects under it, like Rodeo Net in Oregon, which is for mental health case management services, which is what we are funding, and we have a number of other projects like that that are telemedicine.

But the library's projects have tended to be computer-based information sharing systems. The Lister Hill Center at the library, funded a classic telemedicine program, the STARPAC program, which was on the Papago Indian reservations. They demonstrated, using satellite technology, how telemedicine could be used for basically creating protocols and supporting allied health personnel that served on that reservation. It was reasonably successful.

One of the things that we learned from it is the limitations of the technology at that time and the library—I mean, one of the things the library has been very good at, and NIH has been good at, is helping to understand the limitations of the technology. For example, they found that for dermatology consultations, at the time, the technology was not good for people of color. That limited what you could tell about skin infection if you couldn't do it on people with color. That technology has changed rapidly.

Now we can do things we could never think of before now, the technology that we have at the cost people have talked about, less than $50,000, is wonderful for dermatology consultations.

Mrs. MORELLA. It is helpful. You are moving along.

Dr. Sanders, do you avail yourself of any of those services?

Mr. RAVETTO. If I could interject, we operate a learning resource center that is based in Lafayette, Louisiana that is an available to all of our hospitals and facilities—and practitioners within our 13-parish region, and we put Grateful Med in there and the Lonesome Doc, which is excellent, I have to say, and what we did is we realized—we offered an 800 number. We realize there was a step missing.

So what we have done now is we have established a computer network called STAT, it is an acronym for Simple Telephone Access to Technology, where we make available to rural hospitals the hardware and the software, and Dr. Sanders' hospital is one of them. I think it is up to maybe 11 or 12 of our hospitals now have it, so that they can sit down and actually link in directly, and then if they need our library to retrieve anything in hard copy for them, they can do that and it has been extremely successful.

Dr. PUSKIN. You are a part of an area health education center, are you not, which is a program of the Health Resources and Services Administration? AHECs are generally affiliated with medical schools but their purpose is to get out to communities the best that is known for continuing education and keeping people up to date. I think one reason why some of the technology that we have available works better in some areas than others is the active leadership of the AHEC as a focal point for training people on how to use it and being there for consults and technical assistance when practitioners are working with something like Grateful Med or Lonesome Doc, and they want to call someone up and say, "Something is not quite right here."

Mr. RAVETTO. We also use INTERNET too as part of the program.

Dr. RICHARD SANDERS. As a practitioner, I have used Grateful Med, definitely do. However, many of the times what I will do is, I will ask a question to a computer and see if I can get an answer. Because I am in a rural area in family practice, I am not into research, I am not into teaching. Many times I won't go into great detail in reading an article and I will have a question that I will ask, sometimes of practical significance, and see if I can get an answer.

For example, I have a lady who is two months pregnant. She has been exposed to tuberculosis. She has a positive TB skin test. What do we treat her with, questions like that. Somebody who has has had experience with infectious diseases or something.

Mrs. MORELLA. I want to thank the panel. I do remember when I was thinking of you, Dr. Sanders, and the fishing situation and with the crabs and the shrimp and the oysters, when I was in the State legislature, the issue of MSX came up and I thought we don't have a defense budget in Maryland, I don't know why. We would be talking about MSX. MSX is a parasite that oysters get which was a problem in the Chesapeake Bay. The panel has been great, as have all the panels today.

I yield back and thank the Chairman.

Mr. HAYES. With that, we are going to conclude our field hearing and I very much appreciate those of you who have participated, most of whom of you stayed, which believe me, is a very rare experience when you conduct panels, and I think that it enhances to a great deal both those things you might augment in our record for later reading and some of the interchanges that have to lead to better policy and understanding. Thanks again.

With that, we will conclude our Investigations and Oversight Subcommittee hearing on Science, Space and Technology.

[Whereupon, at 2:50 p.m., the subcommittee was adjourned.]

O

81-951 (288)